LEARN MEDICAL TERMINOLOGY

Flash Card Activities, Instructional Videos, & Complete Guide
To Master Medical Terms for Healthcare Professionals

Made by The Medical Professionals of NEDU LLC at NurseEdu.com

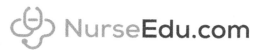 NurseEdu.com

Disclaimer:

Although the author and publisher have made every effort to ensure that the information in this book was correct at press time, the author and publisher do not assume and hereby disclaim any liability to any party for any loss, damage, or disruption caused by errors or omissions, whether such errors or omissions result from negligence, accident, or any other cause.

This book is not intended as a substitute for the medical advice of physicians. The reader should regularly consult a physician in matters relating to his/her health and particularly with respect to any symptoms that may require diagnosis or medical attention.

NCLEX®, NCLEX®-RN, and NCLEX®-PN are registered trademarks of the National Council of State Boards of Nursing, Inc. They hold no affiliation with this product.

Some images within this book are either royalty-free images, used under license from their respective copyright holders, or images that are in the public domain.

ISBN: 978-1-952914-01-0

GET ACCESS CODE

ACCESS BONUS
VIDEOS & FLASH CARDS

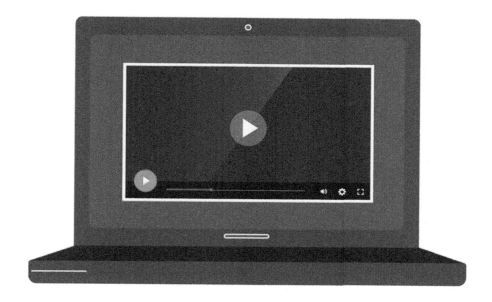

FREE Access With Your Purchase — Just Visit:

nurseedu.com/medterm

TABLE OF CONTENTS

INTRODUCTION TO MEDICAL TERMINOLOGY

Medical terminology involves the—sometimes frustrating and challenging—study of the wide variety of medical terms that underline the sometimes long and complex medical terms used in everyday medical circles. Medical terms are generally created from a combination of prefixes, suffixes, and root words—most of which ultimately originate in the Latin or Greek languages, although some word parts have German, French, or English origins.

This guide should help you learn and understand the different medical word parts that make up medical terminology. There will be medical word parts that are based on numbers, colors, and on Greek and Latin-based prefixes, root words, and suffixes. You'll find some chapters are more complicated because there are a great many word parts to memorize. Others have just a few medical word parts and phrases to memorize. Fear not! Each of these chapters can be mastered.

The first part of this book will involve a barrage of word parts to memorize. Following this, there will be area-specific terms. These will be much easier to swallow once you have learned the root words, prefixes, and suffixes that are laid out in the beginning of the text.

CHAPTER 1:

BASIC WORD ELEMENTS

The best thing about medical terms is that they are mostly based on Greek, Latin, and other terms that, when strung together, create a longer word that makes sense once you know the parts. There are two to four parts to every medical term, which include some combination of the following:

- Root word or term—this is the basic meaning or foundation of the word and often relates to a body part or function.
- Suffix—this is the ending of the word.
- Prefix—this is the beginning of the word.
- Combining vowel—this is a vowel (usually an "o") linking part of the word (such as the root word) to another part (such as the suffix) of the word. It is used to make the word make sense or to make it easier to spell or pronounce.

Word Roots

There are dozens of root words—most of them based on Latin or Greek words. They usually point to a specific body area or to a body function. You may recognize some of them because they are similar to common medical words. These include the following root words:

- Acous—this means "hearing" and is found in words such as "acoustic."
- Acusis—this means "hearing condition" and is found in words such as "hyperacusis," which means exaggerated hearing.
- Aden—this means "gland" and is found in the word "adenopathy," which is a disease of the lymph nodes or lymph "glands."

- Adip—this means "fat" and is found in the term "adipose tissue," which is the medical term for fatty tissue.
- Adrena—this means "adrenal" and refers to the adrenal gland. It can also be modified with a different vowel to make the term "adrenocorticotropic hormone."
- Aer—this means "air" and is found in nonmedical terms, such as aerial, or the medical term "aerophagia," which means "swallowing air."
- Aero—this means "gas" and is used in nonmedical terms, such as aerodynamic or aerospace.
- Albumin—this means "protein" and refers to the most common plasma protein, which is albumin.
- Andr—this stands for "male" and is used to define words like androgenic, which is something originating from the male or "androgen," which is a male hormone.
- Angi—this means "vessel" and is used in cardiovascular terms like "angiogram," which is an X-ray of the blood vessels.
- Aort—this is a root word meaning "aorta," which is the largest artery in the body.
- Arthr—this means "joint" and is used in terms like "arthroscopy," which is a test that involves looking into a joint.
- Audi—this is a term meaning "hearing" and is used in words like "audiogram," which is a hearing test.
- Balan—this is a root word meaning "glans penis" and refers to words like "balanitis," which involves an infection or inflammation of this part of the penis.
- Blephar—this refers to "eyelid." It is used in words like "blepharitis," which is an infection or inflammation of the eyelid.
- Bronch—this is a root word meaning "bronchus." It is used in terms like "bronchial" and "bronchitis," which are words related to the bronchial tree in the lungs.
- Capn—this is a term meaning "carbon dioxide" and is used in terms like "capnography," which is a test that measures the carbon dioxide level in the airway.
- Card—this refers to the "heart" and is used in "cardiology," which is a word meaning the study of the heart.

- Carp—this means "wrist" and relates to terms like "carpal tunnel syndrome," which involves injury to an area around the wrist.

- Cerebr—this is a root word meaning "cerebrum" or brain. The cerebrum is the main "thinking" part of the brain.

- Cerumen—this means "wax-like" or "waxy." The term cerumenectomy refers to removing earwax.

- Chol—this refers to "bile" and is used in terms like "cholecystectomy," which is the removal of the gallbladder, and "cholestasis," which is the stagnation of bile.

- Chondr—this is a term for "cartilage," which is seen in words like "costochondritis," which means an inflammation of the cartilage in the front of the rib cage.

- Col—this means "colon" and is a root word used in "colitis," or inflammation of the colon.

- Cor—this is a term meaning "pupil." It is used in the word "cornea," which covers the pupil.

- Crani—this means "cranium," which is another term for "the skull."

- Cutane—this refers to "skin" and is used in terms like "cutaneous," which means "pertaining to the skin."

- Cyst—this means "bladder" and is used in terms like "cystitis" and "cholecystitis," which are words for bladder inflammation and gallbladder inflammation, respectively.

- Cyt—this means "cell" and is used in words like "erythrocyte," which stands for red blood cell, or "leukocyte," which stands for white blood cell.

- Dacry or Lacrim—this means "tear" or "tear duct." Words like "lacrimation" mean "tearing," and words like "dacryocystitis" refer to inflammation of the tear duct sac.

- Dactyl—this is a term meaning "finger" or "toe." This is used in words like "polydactyly," or "too many" fingers or toes.

- Dementio—this means "to be mad" and is used in the word "dementia," which is a cognitive disorder that occurs in older individuals.

- Derma—this is a root word meaning "skin." Dermatology is the study of skin and skin disorders.

- Duoden—this is a root word for "duodenum," which is the first part of the small intestines.

- Encephal—this means "brain" and is used in medical terms like "encephalopathy" (pathology of the brain) and "electroencephalogram" (or EEG)—an electrical test of the brain.

- Enter—this means "intestine" and is used in "enteritis," or an inflammation of the intestines.

- Esophag—this stands for "esophagus" and is used in medical terms like "esophagoscopy," which is a test of the esophagus.

- Esthesi—this is a word for "sensation" and is used in the medical term "anesthesia," which means a lack of sensation in the body.

- Femor—this means "thigh bone" and is used in terms like "femoral," which refers to arteries, veins, and nerves in the thigh area.

- Fibr—this is a term meaning "fiber." The term "fibrous" involves something that is like fiber.

- Fibul—this means "small, outer, lower leg bone." The fibula is this bone in the human body.

- Gastr—this means "stomach" and is used in terms like "gastritis" (stomach inflammation) and "gastroenterology" (the study of the stomach and the gastrointestinal or "GI" tract).

- Glyc—this means "sugar" and refers to words like "glycogen" (a molecule made of glucose) and "glycolysis" (the breakdown of sugar).

- Gnos—this means recognition or knowledge. It is used in terms like "agnosia," which means the lack of ability to perceive sensory input.

- Gynec—this is a term meaning "woman" and is used in terms like "gynecology" (the study of the female reproductive tract).

- Hemat or Hemo—these mean "blood" and are used in blood-related terms like "hematology" (the study of blood) and "hemolysis" (the breakdown of blood).

- Hepat—this means "liver." "Hepatology" is the study of the liver and "hepatitis" is inflammation of the liver.

- Hist—this means "tissue." "Histology" is the study of tissues.

- Humer—this means "humerus," which is the bone in the upper arm.

- Hyster—this is a term meaning "uterus" and is used to make the words "hysterectomy" (removal of the uterus) and "hysterosalpingogram" (an X-ray study of the tubes and uterus).

- Iri or Irid—these root words mean "iris." "Iritis" is an inflammation of the iris, and "iridectomy" is a surgical excision of the iris.

- Kerat—This root word means "hard" and is used in terms like "keratin," a protein that hardens the skin tissue.

- Lact—this means "milk" and refers to words like "lactase" (an enzyme that digests milk) and "lactation" (which is breastfeeding).

- Lapar—this stands for "abdomen." The word "laparotomy" refers to a surgical procedure in which the abdomen is entered.

- Laryng—this means "larynx," used in the medical term "laryngitis" (an inflammation of the throat or larynx).

- Lipid—this means "fat." In medicine, lipids are another term for fats.

- Lymph—this means "lymph," referring to lymph glands and lymph tissue. "Lymphadenopathy" is an inflammation of the lymph glands.

- Mamm—this is a term for "breast" and helps make words like "mammography" (an X-ray study of the breasts).

- Mast—this means "breast" and is used in the term "mastitis," which is an infection of the breast.

- Mening—this is the medical root word for "meninges." The term "meningitis" is an infection of the meninges.

- Metr—this is a term for "uterus." It is used in the word "endometrium," the inner lining of the uterus.

- My—this is a root word for "muscle" and is used to make words like "myopathy," or a disease of the muscle tissue.

- Myel—this is a root word meaning "spinal cord." A "myelogram" is an X-ray study of the spinal cord.

- Myring—this stands for "eardrum." A "myringotomy" is a surgical procedure involving the use of a surgical instrument to pierce the eardrum.

- Nasal—this means "nose." The nasal bone is a prominent bone in the nose.

- Necr—this means "death" of cells or the body. "Necrosis" is a disease of cell (or tissue death) and "necrophilia" is a desire to have sex with a corpse.

- Nephr—this stands for "kidney" and is used in medical terms like "nephrology" (the study of the kidneys) and "nephritis" (an inflammation of the kidneys).

- Neur—this means "nerve." "Neurology" is the study of the nerves or the nervous system.

- Ocul—this is a term meaning "eye." The "oculomotor nerve" is a nerve that innervates muscles surrounding the eye.

- Onych—this is a word that means "nail." "Onychomycosis" is a fungal infection of the nail.

- Ophthalm—this means "eye." "Ophthalmology" is the study of the eye.

- Orchid or test—these terms mean "testicle" or "testis." "Orchitis" is an inflammation or infection of the testes.

- Oste—this is a term meaning "bone." The word "periosteum" is the covering over the bone tissue.

- Ot—this stands for "ear." The term "otalgia" means pain in the ear.

- Ovari—this is a term for "ovary." An "ovariectomy" is the surgical removal of an ovary.

- Ox—this means "oxygen" and is used in medical terms like "oximetry," which is a test that measures oxygen levels in the body.

- Oxy—this means "oxygen" and is used to make medical terms such as "oxyhemoglobin"—the oxygenated form of the hemoglobin protein.

- Pancreat—this is the term for "pancreas." Pancreatitis is an inflammation or infection of the pancreas.

- Patell—this means "kneecap." In fact, "patella" is the medical term for the kneecap.

- Pector — this is the root word for "chest" and is used do describe the "pectoral muscles," or muscles of the chest wall.

- Ped or pod — this means "foot." A "pedometer" measures a person's steps, while a "podiatrist" is a doctor who studies and treats foot disorders.

- Pelv — this is the term for "pelvis." "Pelvimetry" involves measuring the bones of the pelvis, or the measurement of the pelvic opening.

- Phalang — these are the "bones of fingers and toes," represented by the medical term "phalanges."

- Phleb — this is the term for "vein." The medical term "phlebitis" means an inflammation of the veins.

- Pneum — this means "air" or "lung." "Pneumonia" is an infection in the lungs and "pneumatic" refers to air pressure.

- Prostat — this is the term for "prostate." "Prostatitis" is an infection or inflammation of the prostate gland.

- Pulmon — this means "lung." The term "pulmonary" refers directly to the lungs.

- Ren — this means "kidney" and is used in terms like "renal," which refers to the kidneys.

- Retin — this means "retina." "Retinitis" is an inflammation of the retina or the back of the eye.

- Salping — this is a term meaning "fallopian tube." The term "salpingitis" means an infection of the fallopian tubes. It also means "eustachian tube."

- Sinus — this simply means "sinus" and refers to things like "sinusitis" — an infection of the sinuses.

- Somat — this refers to "body." "Somatic" means anything related to the body.

- Sperm — this means "sperm" and helps make words like "spermatozoa," which are sperm cells.

- Splen — this is the root word for "spleen." A splenectomy is the removal of the spleen.

- Spondy — this is the medical root word for "backbone" or "vertebrae."

"Spondylolisthesis" is a disorder involving slippage of the vertebrae.

- Stenosis—this means "narrowing." "Stenosis" is the medical term referring to a narrowing of a body part or area.

- Stern—this is the medical root word for "sternum" or "breastbone." Surgeons perform a "sternotomy" when they open the chest to do heart surgery.

- Tendin—this means "tendon." The term "tendinitis" means an inflammation of a tendon.

- Thromb—this means "clot." "Thrombophlebitis" is a clot and inflammation inside a vein.

- Thym—this is the medical term for "thymus." The "thymus gland" is located in the superior and anterior part of the upper chest.

- Tibi—this is the root term for "large lower leg bone." The tibia is the largest bone in the lower leg area.

- Toco—this means "birth." The medical term "tocolysis" means to stop the labor or birthing process.

- Tympan—this means "eardrum." The "tympanic membrane" is another word for the eardrum.

- Ureter—this means "ureter." The ureter connects the kidney to the bladder.

- Urethr—this means "urethr," which is the tube that connects the urinary bladder to the outside of the body.

- Uria—this stands for "urination" or "urine." The term "polyuria" means excessive urination.

- Vas—this means "duct" or "vessel." The "vas deferens" is the tube leading out of the testes; it carries sperm cells.

- Vascul—this means "blood vessel." The term "cardiovascular" refers to the heart and blood vessel system.

- Ven—this means "vein." The venous system is the system of the body's veins. "Venography" is an X-ray of the veins.

- Vesic—this means "bladder." The term "vesicular" refers to the bladder. There is also a root word "vesicul," which refers to the seminal vesicles.

Combining Forms

Compared to memorizing all the root words you've just read, learning to combine forms is relatively easy. The combining form of a word is the root word fused with a "combining vowel." In almost all cases, the combining vowel is "o." This letter is used to make it easier to combine root words with other words in the English language. Some examples include the following:

- Aden becomes Aden/o to make words like "adenopathy."
- Arth becomes Arthr/o to make words like "arthroscopy."
- Carcin (which means "cancer") becomes Carcin/o to make words such as "carcinomatosis."
- Cardi becomes Cardi/o to make "cardiology."
- Cephal (which means "head") becomes Cephal/o to make "cephalopelvic."
- Cis (which means "cut") is combined to make "ciso," which is used to make the word "excision" or "to cut out."
- Derm (which means "skin") is combined with "a" to make "dermatology."
- Erythr (which means "red") is combined with "o" to make the word "erythrocyte."
- Gynec becomes Gynec/o to make words like "gynecology."
- Hepat (which means "liver") is combined to make Hepat/o to make "hepatology," or the study of the liver.
- Onc (which means "tumor") combines to make Onc/o for such words as "oncogene" or "oncology."
- Path (which means "disease") combines with "o" to make Path/o and words like "pathology," or the study of disease.
- Radi (which means "X-rays") combines with "o" to make words like "radiology" or the study of X-rays.
- Sarc (which means "flesh") combines to make Sarc/o for the word "sarcoma"—a tumor of the soft tissue.
- Ur (which means "urinary tract") combines with "o" to make words like

"urology" (the study of the urinary tract).

Suffixes

A suffix appears at the end of the root word in medical terms (and other words) and may or may not be affiliated with a prefix. The purpose of a suffix is to amplify or modify the meaning of the word. Some suffixes are used more frequently than others. Let's first start with some of the more common suffixes.

The two most common suffixes in the Greek language are "ia," which in French is "ie" and in English is "y." These suffixes mean "a pathological state or condition." One word used this way is "hysteria," which means a chronic neurosis that used to be thought of as being uterine in origin.

The suffix "iasis" means a pathological state, such as "lithiasis," which means the formation of stones or urinary calculi, and "psoriasis," which means a pathological skin disease.

The endings "ikos," "icus," or "ic" (in English) connotes an adjective. The term "anesthetic" means referring to, or pertaining to, anesthesia. The term "epileptic" refers to epilepsy.

The terms "ismos" or "ismus" or "ism" denote some type of condition. The term "embolism" means the plugging of an artery or vein, while "hypnotism" is a condition of artificially-caused sleep.

The suffix "istis" or "ist" (in English) means a doer or agent of an action. A "hypnotist" is the agent who causes "hypnosis" in an individual. The "anesthetist" delivers anesthesia.

The suffix "itis" means a disease state or inflammation. It forms multiple inflammatory words like "arthritis," "bursitis," and "conjunctivitis."

The suffix "ize" means treatment using a special instrument or drug. One word used with this suffix is "hypnotize," which means to put to sleep or into a hypnotic state.

The suffixes "ma" or "ema" or "oma" mean a specific pathological condition. There are a number of words ending in "oma," which usually indicate some type of pathological tumor. "Carcinoma" is a cancerous tumor and a "granuloma" is a tumor of granulation tissue.

The suffix "oid" was originally "oeid," which means the form or appearance of something that resembles something else. "Sphenoid" means wedge-shaped as "sphen" means wedge. "Typhoid" means related to "typhus fever."

The suffix "sis" or "osis" means any production or increase in something. It can be used interchangeably with "iasis." "Tuberculosis" means an invasion of the tubercle bacillus.

The chemical suffix "ase," which means a substance is an enzyme. This applies to words like "lipase" and "amylase," which are both enzymes.

The suffix "ate" means the salt of a base. One word made from this is "phosphate," which is the salt of phosphoric acid, and "sulphate," which is the salt of "sulfuric acid."

The suffix "ide" is the name for a binary compound containing a nonmetal element, such as "chloride" or "iodide." The suffix "in" denotes a termination of a glucoside, as in "fibrin" and "gelatin."

The suffix "ine" refers to an ending used to name alkaloids. "Morphine" is the alkaloid of opium.

The suffix "ite" is the term used to indicate the salt of some type of acid. A salt of phosphorus is "phosphite," while "sulphite" is a salt of sulfurous acid.

These are some less commonly used Greek suffixes:

- **Agogue.** This comes from the Greek word "agogos," which means leader. A "galactagogue" is something that promotes the secretion of milk, and a "hypnagogue" is an inducer of sleep.
- **Agra.** This means seizure. A "cardiagra" is a heart seizure, another name for angina pectoris.
- **Algia.** This means pain. The medical term "myalgia" means muscle pain, and "arthralgia" means joint pain.
- **Asthenia.** This comes from the Greek word "asthenes," which means weak. "Neurasthenia" means nerve weakness or nervous exhaustion.
- **Cele.** This comes from the Greek word "kele." It means tumor, hernia, or protrusion. "Hematocele" means blood cyst, and "hydrocele" means water hernia.
- **Cinesia.** This comes from the Greek word "kinesis," which means movement. "Enterocinesia" means movement of the intestines.

- **Clasia or Clasis.** These words mean breaking. The word "arthroclasia" means the breaking of a joint or breaking up of adhesions.

- **Cyte or Kytos.** These words mean cell. "Erythrocyte" is the name for a red blood cell and "leukocyte" is a white blood cell.

- **Ectomy.** This means excision. A "hysterectomy" means the excision of the uterus, while a "thyroidectomy" is the excision of the thyroid gland.

- **Ectopia.** This means out of place. The term "nephrectopia" means an abnormal mobility of the kidney, while "splenectopia" means an abnormal mobility of the spleen.

- **Emia.** This means blood. It is used in medical terms such as "hyperemia," which means an increase in blood or an increase in blood flow.

- **Esthesia.** This means feeling or sensibility. "Paresthesia" is a medical term that means an abnormal sensation.

- **Genesis.** This means generation or origin. This is used in the word "pathogenesis," which is the origin or development of a disease state.

- **Graphy.** This is from the word "graphein," which means to write. "Ventriculography" is a radiograph of the cerebral ventricles.

- **Lith.** This is a Greek word meaning stone. An "enterolith" is an intestinal stone or intestinal calculus.

- **Logia or Logie.** This comes from the Greek word "logos," which means treatise, discourse, or word. "Physiology" is the study which deals with life processes. "Urology" is the study of diseases of the urinary organs. The suffix "logy" is a natural anglicizing of the word "logie."

- **Lysis.** This means loosening or dissolution. The term "hemolysis" means the breakdown or dissolution of red blood cells.

- **Macia.** This comes from the Greek word "malakia," which means the softening of muscular tissues. "Osteomalacia" is softening of the bones, for example.

- **Mania.** This means having an uncontrollable impulse or madness. "Kleptomania" means having a pathological impulse to steal things.

- **Megaly.** This comes from the Greek word "megas," which means large.

"Acromegaly" is an enlargement of the bones of the extremities, while "splenomegaly" is an enlargement of the spleen.

- **Odynia.** This is a Greek word meaning pain. "Acrodynia" is a pain in the extremities, while "otodynia" is a pain in the ear.

- **Opia.** This means vision. "Amblyopia" is a dimness of vision (as "amblys" means dull).

- **Pathy.** This comes from the Greek word "pathos," which means suffering. "Adenopathy" is the medical term meaning glandular disease.

- **Philia.** This comes from the Greek word "philein." It means to like. "Hemophilia" roughly means the "liking of blood," which is actually a blood disorder.

- **Phobia.** This comes from the Greek word "phobos." Simply put, it means fear. "Claustrophobia" is a morbid fear of being in an enclosed space.

- **Plasty.** This comes from the Greek term "plassein," which means to form. "Enteroplasty" is plastic surgery of the intestines.

- **Plegia.** This comes from the Greek word "pleg," which means stroke. "Hemiplegia" is a "half stroke" or paralysis of one side of the body.

- **Poeisis.** This is a Greek suffix meaning to form or make. "Hematopoiesis" is the formation of blood.

- **Pyosis.** This comes from the Greek word "pyon," which means pus. The word "arthropyosis" means pus or suppuration of a joint.

- **Rrhagia.** This also forms the suffix "-rrhage," which means to break forth. "Hemorrhage" literally means bleeding, while "metrorrhagia" means excessive bleeding of the uterus.

- **Rrhaphy.** This means "stitch." The term "perineorrhaphy" refers to suturing of the perineum.

- **Rhea.** This means "flow." "Gonorrhea" means a discharge or "flow" coming from the gonococcus organism.

- **Sclerosis.** This means hardening. It forms the word "arteriosclerosis," which is a hardening of the arteries.

- **Scope.** This is related to the suffix "scopy," which means to view. "Cystoscopy" is the viewing of the inside of the bladder.

- **Spasm.** This comes from the Greek word "spasmos," which means a cramp or convulsion. An "enterospasm" is another name for intestinal colic, while "pylorospasm" is a painful contraction of the pylorus.

- **Staxis.** This means oozing, dripping, or a slow hemorrhage. Epistaxis means "nose bleed" and uses this term as its suffix.

- **Stomy.** This comes from the Greek word "stoma," which means mouth. A "colostomy" is the forming of an opening or "mouth" out of the intestinal tract.

- **Therapy.** This comes from the Greek word "therapeia," which means treatment. "Hydrotherapy" literally means water treatment or water therapy.

- **Thermy.** This comes from the Greek word meaning heat. "Diathermy" involves increasing the temperature by an electric current.

- **Tomy.** This means an incision into something. A "lobotomy" is an operation on the frontal lobe.

- **Troph.** This means "to nourish." "Atrophy" is a medical term that means a lack of nourishment, or a wasting of the tissues of the body. "Hypertrophy" means excessive nourishment or overgrowth.

- **Uria.** This is a Greek suffix meaning to urinate. "Hematuria" means "blood in the urine."

There are a number of typical suffixes that come directly from the Latin language. Here are a few:

- **Ago or igo.** This comes from the Latin word for drive. It suggests activity. "Lumbago" is a rheumatism of the lumbar region. "Vertigo" is giddiness or dizziness and comes from the Latin word "vertere," which means to turn around.

- **Algis.** This also can be "al," which is an adjectival suffix. For example, the word "crucial" means decisive, and "digital" means relating to or resembling a digit.

- **Culum.** This is "cle" in English and means a little body. For example, the term "follicle" means little bag, and "ventricle" means little belly.

- **Or.** This denotes an agent or state. A "donor" is, for example, a giver, which comes from the Latin word "donare" ("to give"). The term "levator" is one that lifts, which comes from the Latin word "levare" ("to lift").

- **Orium.** This is a designation of a space, such as a "sanitorium," which is a place for treatment. "Tentorium" means an anatomical part that resembles a covering or tent.

- **Osus.** This translates into "ous" or "ose" in English and represents an adjectival suffix. The term "aqueous" basically means watery. The term "adipose" means fatty.

- **Tas or Ty.** This denotes an abstract quality or idea. It is used in the term "acidity," which is the state of being acid. "Immunity" is the resistance to disease states.

- **Tio or Tion.** This is a suffix that basically means an action or function. For example, "inflammation" involves a morbid change in the body's tissues. "Palpation" is an examination performed by using the hands.

Prefixes

The most important prefixes come from the Greek language. One major ones is "a" or "an,"which is a negative prefix; it conveys a lack of something, a weakness, or a deficiency. This prefix helps form the medical and nonmedical terms "apathy," which means a lack of feelings, "anemia," which means a lack of blood, and "anesthesia," which means a lack of sensation.

Another common prefix is "amphi" or "ampho," which means on both sides. It can be used to make the words "amphibious," which means living on both sides of land and water, or "amphitheater," which means a place for seeing a show.

The prefix "ana" means up, upward, or again. It forms the words "analysis," which means the breaking up a chemical compound, "anatomy," which means cutting up or dissection, and "anaphylaxis."

The term "anti" means against or opposed to. An "antidote" is a substance that acts against something else (like a poison), while an "antipyretic" is something that fights fever.

The prefix "apo" means off, away from. "Apostaxis," for example, means a slight hemorrhage or trickling of blood.

The Greek prefix "cata" means down or downward. "Catatonia" means a downward tone or stupor, and "catarrha" means a flowing down or an inflammation of the mucus membranes.

The prefix "dia" means through or across, and it forms words like "diabetes," which means to siphon or to go through. "Diarrhea" means to flow through or have a liquid discharge. "Diagnosis" means knowing completely the nature of a disease state.

"Dys" means bad, defective, or difficult. It forms words like "dysentery," which means bad intestine, and "dyspepsia," which means bad digestion. "Dyspnea" means to have difficulty breathing.

The prefixes "ec" or "ex" mean out, outward, or out of. They form words such as "ectopic," which means "out of place," and "eczema," which means a boiling out. "Exophthalmos" means a bulging out of the eye, and "exostosis" means a bony tumor outside of the bone.

"Em" and "en" mean in or within. These form words like "embolism," which means thrown in, or the plugging of a blood vessel.

"Hyper" means above, over, or excessive. It forms "hyperemia," which means excessive blood, and "hyperthyroidism," which means an overactive thyroid gland. "Hypo" is the opposite of "hyper" and means under, insufficient, or below. The term "hypodermic" means under the skin.

"Meta" means after, beyond, change, or behind. It forms the terms "metamorphosis," which means a change in form of something, and "metabolism," which means change in throwing, or tissue change.

"Para" means alongside, near, or apart from. The term "paranoia" means abnormal in the mind.

"Peri" means about or around. The "pericardium" is the covering layer around the heart, and "periosteum" is the covering around the bone.

"Pro" means before, in advance, or forward. The term "prodrome" means an early symptom, or "running before." "Prophylaxis" means advanced protection.

The prefixes "syn" or "sym" mean with or together. The medical term "symbiosis" means two or more organisms living together. "Symptom" means a falling together or a sign.

There are some very common Greek-based adverbs that act as prefixes to numerous medical terms. Some of these include:

- **Di.** This means "twice" and is used in terms like "diploid," which means having twice the number of chromosomes.

- **Endo.** This means within and is used in terms like "endocrine," which means secretion within the body, and "endometrium," which means the lining within the uterus.

- **Eu.** This means "well" or "easy" and is used in terms like "euthanasia," which means "easy death."

- **Exo.** This means "outside" or "outward" and is used in terms like "exogenous," meaning originating outside of something.

- **Opisth.** This means behind. It is used in terms like "opisthotonos," which refers to stretching backward, as in a tetanic spasm.

- **Palin.** This means backward, again, or back, and is used in terms like "palindrome," which is a word that reads the same backward and forward.

- **Tele.** This means distant and is used in terms like "telescope," which refers to a device that can see long distances.

Similar to Greek prefixes, there are Latin prefixes that, when connected to a stem, will change the meaning of the word. Sometimes the consonant at the end of the prefix will change so that it sounds better in the final product. For example, the prefix "ad" becomes "as" for the word "assume." The most important Latin prefixes are listed here:

- **A or Ab or Abs.** These mean off or away from. The term "avulsion" means a tearing away of something, while "abductor" means leading away from the body.

- **Ad.** This is a prefix meaning "to." The word "adhesion" means sticking to, while "adrenal" means near the kidney, which describes the adrenal gland's location.

- **Ambi or ambo.** Thesemean both or on both sides. The term "ambidextrous" means being able to use both hands, and "ambosexual" means bisexual or affecting both sexes.

- **Ante.** This means before in space or time, in front of, or forward. The term "antecubital" means before the elbow, and "anteflexion" means bending forward. "Antenatal" means before birth.

- **Bi or bis.** These mean double or twice. The term "bicarbonate" means a salt having two molecules of carbonic acid, and "bicuspid" means having two points.

- **Circum.** This means around. "Circumcision" means cutting around. The term "circumocular" means around the eye, while "circumoral" means around the mouth.

- **Con or co.** These mean with or together. The word "coagulation" means the formation of clots. The term "concussion" means a violent shock.

- **Contra.** This means opposed to or against. "Contraception" means something that is against conception.

- **De.** This means down or downward. This makes words like "decompensation," which means putrefaction or decay, while "dementia" means without mind.

- **Di or Dis.** These mean apart or negative. It helps form the word "dissect," which means to cut apart, and "digestion," which means carrying food away.

- **E or Ec or Ex.** These prefixes mean out, removal, off, or out of. The word "ejection" means the act of throwing out. The word "enucleate" means to remove whole. "Exudate" means to sweat out or sweat.

- **Extra or extro.** These prefixes mean outside of, or outer side. The term "extracellular" refers to outside of the cell, while "extravasation" means a release or loss of blood from a vessel into the tissues.

- **Im.** This means inside, into, or in. It helps form the word "immersion," which means placing a body under water.

- **In or Im.** These prefixes mean "negation." They help form the word "inseparable," which means unable to be separated, and "immaculate," which means without a blemish.

- **Infra.** This means "below" or "beneath." The word "infraorbital" means below the eye. The word "infrared" means beyond the red end of the light spectrum.

- **Inter.** This is a prefix meaning "between." The term "intercellular" means between cells, and the term "interdigital" means between the fingers or toes.

- **Intra.** This prefix means within or inside of. The word "intracellular" means within the cell, and "intravenous" means within a vein.

- **Juxta.** This means near or beside. "Juxta-articular" means situated near a joint.

- **Ob.** This prefix means in front of, near, or against. The word "obliteration" means complete removal, while "obstetrics" literally means to stand in front of a woman. The term "occlusion" actually originates from "obclusion," but the "b" has been replaced by a "c" as per Latin custom. It means the act of closure or the state of being closed.

- **Per.** This means thorough, very, or excessive. "Percutaneous" means through the skin. "Permeable" means permitting a passage through.

- **Post.** This means behind, after, or following. The term "post-febrile" means after fever, and "postpartum" means after birth.

- **Pre.** This means before, in front of, or anterior. "Prefrontal" is the medical anatomic term for the part of the cortex that is most anterior. "Productive" means leading forward, capable of producing. "Prolapse" means to sink, or fall forward.

- **Re.** This means back or again. The term "reduce" means to lead back.

- **Retro.** This is an anatomic prefix, which means backward or back. The term "retroflexion" means bending backward, while "retrograde" means going backward or moving backward.

- **Sub or sup.** These mean below, beneath, or downward. The medical term "subliminal" means below the threshold of sensation.

- **Super or supra.** These mean above. "Superciliary" means above the eyebrow. "Supra-costal" means above the rib, and "suprapubic" means above the pubic arch.

- **Trans.** This means through, across, or beyond. The term "transference" means to carry across, while "transfusion" means pouring across or the process of transferring blood.

- **Ultra.** This means beyond or in excess. "Ultrafiltration" means extra-fine filtration. Ultraviolet rays are light rays beyond the violet spectrum.

- **Ilio.** This comes from the verb, ilium, which means "flank." The medical term "iliocostal" relates to both the flank and the ribs.

- **Latus.** This means side and is used in the medical term "lateral," which refers to the side of something. "Lateroflexion" refers to bending or curvature to the side.

- **Albus.** This means white and starts words like "alboferrin," which is a light brown iron powder.

- **Anter.** This is a shortened way of saying "anterior," which means "in front of." The word "anterograde" means moving forward. "Anterolateral" means anterior and in front of.

- **Dextro.** This means right. Dextromanual is the medical term for being right-handed.

- **Mal.** This comes from the Latin word "malus," which means bad or evil. It helps form the word "maladjustment," which means poor adjustment. The term "malpractice" means the mistreatment of a disease.

- **Medio.** This comes from the Latin word "medius," which means middle. "Mediolateral" is a medical term, which means in the middle and to one side.

- **Multi.** This comes from the Latin term "multus," which means many. "Multiform" is a medical term that means "occurring in many forms." A "multigravida" is a woman who has had more than one child.

- **Pluri.** This comes from the Latin word "plus." It helps form words like "pluriglandular," which involves several different glands or their secretions.

- **Primi.** This comes from the Latin term "primus," which means first. "Primipara" refers to a woman giving birth for the first time.

- **Postero.** This comes from the Latin term "posterior," which means behind. The word "posterolateral" refers to something behind and to the side.

- **Semi.** This is a Latin term meaning part or half. A person who is "semicomatose" is someone who exhibits some, but not all, symptoms of a coma.

- **Sinister or sinistro.** These are Latin for left. Something that is "sinistrocerebral" refers to the left side of the cerebrum or brain.

- **Uni.** This comes from the Latin word "unus," which means one. Uniaxial is something that has just one axis. Something that is "unilateral" has just one side.

- **Form.** This comes from the Latin term "forma," which means form or shape. The term "cuneiform" is something that is "wedge-shaped." Something that is "fusiform" is spindle-shaped.

- **Fuge.** This comes from the Latin word "fugare," which means to drive away or expel. A "centrifuge" is an apparatus that drives microscopic particles to the center.

- **A-. an-.** These prefixes refer to "not" or "without" and are used in words such as "anile," which means of (or like) a foolish, doddering old woman.

- **Anti-.** This is a negative prefix referring to "against." It is used in words such as "antithesis," which means opposition or contrast, as in the antithesis of right and wrong.

- **Contra-.** This is a negative prefix referring to "against." It is used in words such as "contraband," which means anything prohibited by law from being imported or exported.

- **De-.** This prefix refers to "down" or "without." It is used in words like "deinstitutionalize," which means to release (a person with mental or physical disabilities) from a hospital, asylum, home, or other institution.

- **Dis-.** This prefix refers to "absent, removal, or separation" and is a negative prefix used in words such as "disavow," which means to disclaim knowledge of, connection with, or responsibility for, to disown, to repudiate.

- **Olig/o-.** This prefix means "few" or "scanty" and is a prefix indicating the degree of something. It is used in words such as "oligomenorrhea" and means abnormally infrequent menstruation or abnormally scanty blood flow in menstruation.

- **Pan-.** This prefix means "all" and is a prefix indicating the degree of something. It is used in words such as "panhypopituitarism," which means the entire pituitary gland is hypo-functioning.

- **Super-.** This prefix means "excess" or "above" and can be a prefix showing the degree of something or the position of something. It is used in words such as "superfluous," which means being more than is sufficient or required, excessive.

- **Eu-.** This is a prefix meaning "true," "good," "easy," or "normal". It is a prefix used to define size and comparison and is used in words like "euphemism," which means the substitution of a mild, indirect, or vague expression for one thought to be offensive, harsh, or blunt.

- **Hetero-.** This is a prefix meaning "other," "different," or "unequal." It is often a prefix used for size and comparison. It is used in words such as "heterosexual," meaning pertaining to the opposite sex or to both sexes.

- **Homo- or Homeo-.** These prefixes mean "same" or "unchanging" and are prefixes relating to size and comparison. They are used in words such as "homeopathy," which means the method of treating disease by drugs (given in minute doses) that would produce, in a healthy person, symptoms similar to those of the disease (as opposed to allopathy).

- **Iso-.** This prefix means "equal" or "same" and defines the size of something or compares something. It is used in words such as "isometric," which means of (or relating to) isometric exercise.

- **Macro-.** This prefix means "large" or "abnormally large." It is a prefix that indicates size and comparison and is used in words such as "macrosomia," which means an abnormally large size of the body.

- **Mega-.** This prefix means "large" or "abnormally large." It can also mean "one million." It is a prefix used to indicate size or comparison and is used in words like "megalomania," which means an obsession with doing extravagant or grand things.

- **Megalo-.** This prefix means "large" or "abnormally large." It is a prefix used to indicate size and comparison. It is used in words like "megalomania," which means (in psychiatry) a symptom of mental illness marked by delusions of greatness, wealth, etc.

- **Micro-.** This prefix means "small," but it can also mean "one millionth." It is a prefix that measures size and comparison and is used in terms such as "microscope." A microscope is an optical instrument that has a magnifying lens, or a combination of lenses, for inspecting objects too small to be seen by the unaided eye.

- **Neo-.** This is a prefix meaning "new" and is often used to indicate size and comparison. An example is the word "neophyte," which means a beginner or novice.

- **Normo-.** This is a prefix meaning "normal" and is often used to indicate size and comparison. It is used in words such as "normocytic," which means an erythrocyte of normal size.

- **Ortho-.** This is a prefix meaning "straight" or "connected." It is a prefix used to indicate size and comparison. It is used in words such as "orthopedics," which is the medical specialty concerned with deformities or functional impairments of the skeletal system.

- **Poikilo-.** This is a prefix meaning "varied" or "irregular." It is a prefix used to indicate comparison or size. It is used in words like "poikilocytosis," which means the presence of poikilocytes (cells of varying sizes) in the peripheral blood.

- **Pseudo-.** This is a prefix meaning "false" and is used to indicate size and comparison. It is used in words such as "pseudomembranous," which means relating to (or marked by) a false membrane.

- **Re-.** This prefix refers to "again" or "back" and is used to indicate size and comparison. It is used in words such as "reanimate," which means to restore to life or to resuscitate.

- **Ante-.** This prefix refers to "before" and is a prefix of time and/or position. It is used in words such as "antemortem," which means before death, as in an antemortem confession.

- **Pre-.** This prefix refers to "before" or "in front of" and it indicates time and/or position. It is used in words such as "preface," which means something preliminary or introductory.

- **Pro-.** This prefix refers to "before" or "in front of" and it indicates time and/or position. It is used in words such as "pro forma," which means according to form, as a matter of form, for the sake of form.

- **Post-.** This prefix refers to "after" or "behind" and it indicates time and/or position. It is used in words such as "postmortem," which means of, relating to, or occurring in the time following death.

- **Dextr/o-.** This prefix means "right" and it indicates position. It is used in terms such as "dextrorotatory," which is used in optics; it means turning to the right, as the rotation to the right of the plane of polarization of light in certain crystals and the like.

- **Sinistr/o-.** This prefix means "left" and it defines the position of things. It is used in words such as "sinistrodextral," which means moving or extending from the left to the right.

- **Ec-.** This prefix means "out" or "outside" and it indicates the position of things. It is used in words such as "ectoplasm," which means the outer portion of the cytoplasm of a cell.

- **Ecto-.** This prefix means "out" or "outside" and it indicates the position of things. It is used in words such as "ectomere," which means (in biology) any of the blastomeres that participate in the development of the ectoderm.

- **Ex/o-.** This prefix means "away from" or "outside" and it refers to the position of something. An example of a word using exo is "exosphere," which means the highest region of the atmosphere.

- **End/o-.** This is a prefix that means "in" or "within" and it indicates position. It is used in words such as "endoskeleton," which means (in zoology) the internal skeleton or framework of the body of an animal (as opposed to exoskeleton).

- **Mes/o-.** This prefix means "middle" and is used to indicate the position of things. An example of a word with this prefix is "mesoderm," which means (in embryology) the middle germ layer of a metazoan embryo.

- **Syn-.** This prefix means "together" and it indicates the position of things. It is used in words like "synergy," which means (in medicine) the cooperative action of two or more muscles, nerves, or the like.

- **Sym-.** This is a prefix meaning "together" and is often used before "b," "m," or "p." It is a prefix indicating the position of things. An example of a word with this prefix is "symbiosis," which means (in psychiatry) a relationship between two people in which each person is dependent upon and receives reinforcement from the other. In biology, it refers to the living together of two dissimilar organisms, as in mutualism, commensalism, amensalism, or parasitism.

- **Tel/o-.** This prefix means "end" and it indicates the position of things. It is used in terms such as "telomere," which means the segment of DNA that occurs at the ends of chromosomes.

- **Tel/e-.** This prefix means "end" and it indicates the position of things. It is used in words such as "telescope," which is an optical instrument that makes distant objects appear larger and nearer.

Terms related to Color

These are the prefixes often used to describe the color of things:

- **Melan-.** This prefix means "black" and refers to the color black. It is used in the medical term "melanoma," which means any of several types of skin tumors characterized by the cancerous growth of melanocytes.

- **Leuk-.** This prefix means "white" and refers to the color white. It is used in the medical term "leukocyte," which means white blood cell.

- **Poli-.** This prefix means "gray" and refers to the color gray. It is used in the medical term "poliomyelitis" and means an acute viral disease, characterized by inflammation of the motor neurons of the brain stem and spinal cord, which results in motor paralysis.

- **Erythr-.** This prefix means "red" and refers to the color red. It is used in the medical term "erythrocyte," which means red blood cell.

- **Rub(e), Rubr-.** This prefix means "red" and refers to the color red. It is used in the medical term "rubric," which means written, inscribed in, or marked with the color red.

- **Chlor-.** This prefix means "green" and refers to the color green. It is used in the biological term "chlorophyll," which is the green coloring matter of leaves and plants.

- **Cyan-.** This prefix means "blue" and refers to the color blue. It is used in the medical term "cyanosis," which means blueness of the skin, as from poorly oxygenated blood.

- **Xanth-** This prefix means "yellow" and refers to the color yellow. It is used in the medical term "xanthoma," which means a yellow papule or nodule in the skin, containing lipid deposits.

- **Chromo-.** This prefix means "color" and refers to any color. It is used in the word "chromatography," which is a chemistry term meaning the separation of mixtures into their constituents by color.

- **Cirrhos-.** This prefix refers to "yellow" and refers to the color yellow. It is used in the medical term "cirrhosis," which means yellowing of the skin due to a disease of the liver.

- **Luteu-.** This means "yellow" and refers to the color yellow. In medical terms, it is used in the phrase "corpus luteum," which refers to a yellow cyst on the body of the ovary.

- **Porphyro-.** This prefix means "purple" and refers to the color purple. It is used in the medical term "porphyria," which means a defect of blood pigment metabolism in which porphyrins are produced in excess and are found in the urine.

- **Tephr poli-.** This prefix means "gray" and refers to being ashen or gray. It is used to describe someone who has an ashen gray color.

- **Fuchs-.** This prefix refers to "dark brown" and refers to a dark brown color. It is used in the word "fuchsia," where it means a plant belonging to the genus Fuchsia, of the evening primrose family.

- **Glauc-.** This prefix refers to "gray" or "bluish green" and refers to these colors. It is used in medical terminology in the word "glaucoma," which means abnormally high fluid pressure in the eye.

Now that you know so many root words, suffixes, and prefixes, you can use this knowledge to put together (and understand) the meaning of any type of medical term. In later chapters, we'll separate the different medical terms by the area of the body they come from. You'll be much better able to understand their meaning thanks to the understanding you gained in this chapter.

CHAPTER 2:

RULES TO DEFINING AND BUILDING MEDICAL TERMINOLOGY

You've already studied a dizzying number of medical prefixes, suffixes, combining forms, and root words. So how do you use these to define what a word in medicine means? Here's something to consider that's even more complicated: can you build a word that actually means something based on what you know? It turns out there are rules and steps to follow that will help you to know both what a word means and how to build a medical term based on the different parts of that word. As you'll see, defining words is relatively easy, while actually building them can be more complicated.

The 3 Steps Defining Medical Terminology

Let's say you are faced with either the term "poikilocytosis" or "agnosia." These are uncommon medical terms that can trip up even the best of medical professionals. How do you understand what they mean? Let's look at the steps required to define these terms:

Step One: Define the Suffix First

Why the suffix first? Suffixes are relatively easy to figure out and will help you to understand what kind of term you are dealing with. For example, with poikilocytosis, you know that thesuffix is "osis," which means you are dealing with "any production or increase in something." Whatever the term means, you are dealing with an "excess of something." In the case of agnosia, the suffix is "ia," which means you are dealing with "a pathological state or condition." Theis is a good start to knowing what these terms are all about.

Step Two: Define the First Part of the Word

The first part of the word can be a prefix, a combining form, or a root word. In the case of poikilocytosis, you can identify a prefix known as "poikilo," which means "varied" or "irregular." So far, you know that the term means an excess of something that is irregular.

In agnosia, you find the prefix "a," which indicates a lack of something, a weakness, or a deficiency in something. You know so far that this word means a pathological state or condition in which there is a lack of, or deficiency, in something. This naturally leads to wondering what the root words are, which will fully define the word.

Step Three: Define the Root Word

The root word tells you the area of the body, or the area of medicine, being discussed. It is the "aha" moment when you finally put together the meaning of the word. In poikilocytosis, you have the root word "cyt" which means cell. Now you know that the word means "an excess or increase in production of irregular cells." This refers to hematology, in which the word is a nonspecific term for variation in red blood cell shape.

Looking at agnosia, you see the root word "gnos" which means "recognition or knowledge." Putting it all together, you see that agnosia must mean a condition involving the lack of ability to know or recognize something. The definition in medicine is "the inability to process sensory information." Often, this involves the loss of ability to recognize objects, persons, sounds, shapes, or smells despite normal sensory input. You may not have gotten the definition perfectly from putting together the actual "medical terminology meaning," but you've gotten close enough to have a basic understanding of it.

Let's put together a few more words so you get the hang of it:

Hemigastrectomy

This can be split up into "hemi/gastr/ectomy." The suffix means the removal of something, while hemi means half of something. You recognize that "gastr" means "related to the stomach" so the whole term means "removal of half of the stomach."

Bipedal

This can be split into "bi/ped/al." The suffix is "al," which means "of or pertaining to." The prefix "bi" means "two" of something. You recognize that "ped" means foot or feet. Put together, means "pertaining to two feet." In medicine and anthropology, the term means "anything that moves with two legs."

Quadriplegia

This can be split into "quadr/i/plegia." This term is a bit more complex because it has a combining vowel form in the middle. The suffix "plegia" means "stroke or paralysis." The prefix means "four." In this case, the combining vowel is "i". Combined, it means "stroke or paralysis of four of something." In medicine, this term refers to paralysis of all four extremities, usually from a cervical spine injury.

Hemochromatosis

This can be broken into "hemo/chromat/osis." The suffix means "an excess of something." In this case, the classical prefix "chromo" is in the middle of the word and has "at" instead of the "o" vowel, but you can still recognize it as pertaining to color. "Hemo" relates to the blood system and heme ("the deep red-pigmented, iron-containing prosthetic group of hemoglobin and myoglobin"), as you'll soon find out. So, you can work out that this term involves an excess of something related to the colored pigment in blood. The actual medical term means "an inherited disorder characterized by an abnormally high absorption of iron by the intestinal tract, resulting in excessive storage of iron." Again, you may not have worked out the exact definition of hemochromatosis, but you've come close.

Endoscopic Retrograde Cholangiopancreatography

This is a long and convoluted term that often goes by the acronym "ERCP." Let's tackle this one. First, look at "endoscopic," which can be divided into endo/scop/ic. The suffix means "pertaining to," the prefix means "in or within," and the root word "scop" means "to view." Put together, this means "pertaining to viewing something within." Let's look at the second word, "retrograde." This is divided to make retro/grade. The suffix means "pass gradually from one level into another," while the prefix means "back or backward." Put together, this means "to pass something backward" or "going backward." Finally, there is the long word "cholangiopancreatography." This is easily disassembled to make chol/angi/o/pancreat/o/graphy. "Chol" means bile, "angi" means vessel, "pancreat" means pancreas, and "graphy" means "to write." In medicine, the term usually means "to study or record." When these parts are combined, it means to record or study the bile ducts and pancreas. Putting it all together, you get this definition: an internal viewing study that looks backward at the pancreas and bile ducts. This is, in fact, basically what the term really means. The actual definition is "a diagnostic procedure done to look for diseases of the bile ducts and pancreas."

The 9 Rules to Building Medical Terminology

Can you really use medical prefixes, suffixes, and root words that will make sense to other medical personnel? Well, this is more difficult, and it would be easy to get this wrong because there are often prefixes and suffixes that are different but mean the same thing. Even so, you can get close enough to have the word make sense.

These are nine basic rules you need to follow:

Rule Number One

In general, when using more than one root word (as in a compound word like cholangiopancreatography), you need to use a combining vowel in order to separate the different word roots—even if the second or third root word begins with a vowel (although there are exceptions). For example, in "chol/angi," there are two root words that are connected without a combining vowel. When looking at "angi/o/pancreat," however, you see there is a combining vowel (the letter "o"). With "pancreat/o/graphy,"there is also a combining vowel.

Rule Number Two

A word cannot end with a combining form/vowel. This is only done in slang as in "sending the patient to the angio lab." The word "angi/o" doesn't exist as a real medical term; it must have a suffix added to it. A combining vowel must be used if the suffix begins with a consonant, but it is generally not used if the suffix begins with a vowel. In the case of "angio," the suffix is "gram" to make the word "angi/o/gram" or angiogram: "an X-ray photograph of blood or lymph vessels."

Rule Number Three

If the suffix begins with a vowel, the root word can attach directly to it. If, however, the suffix begins with a consonant (any letter in the alphabet other than "a," "e," "i," "o," "u," "y"), the root word will require a combining vowel before attaching to the suffix. What about the word "hematology"? It can be broken into these medical terms: "hemat/o/logy." The suffix starts with a consonant and the root word ends with a consonant, so it needs a combining vowel. Usually, this is "o."

A more difficult word, "hypochondriasis," breaks down like this: "hypo/chondr/iasis." Just so you know, the medical term doesn't mean anything close to what the word looks like it should mean. In any event, "iasis" means "a pathological condition" and "chondr" means cartilage. Since the suffix begins with a vowel, no combining vowel is necessary. However, it doesn't mean "a pathological condition where there is something under the cartilage." Instead, it means "having a morbid concern about one's health." Go figure.

Rule Number Four

Prefixes, of which there are dozens, are (almost always) placed at the beginning of the word. If building a medical term from scratch, you'd need to know if the word needed a prefix and what that prefix should be. Consider trying to make a word meaning "before death." Would you use the prefix "pre" or "ante"? Both "pre" and "ante" mean "before."

Is it "premortem" or "antemortem"? As it turns out, both are real words but, in medicine, the term "antemortem" is more commonly used.

One exception we've already talked about is "hemochromatosis." The prefix "chromo," meaning "color," is attached to the middle of the word rather than the beginning of the word. This is a rare finding and for the most part you can safely assume that, if the word has a prefix, it will be at the beginning of the word.

Rule Number Five

A suffix needs to be placed at the end of the word root. You'll probably find that most medical terms will have a suffix, whereas prefixes are not always necessary. One exception might be the word "anesthesia," which means "lack of sensation." The word breaks up into this: "an/esthesia" or "an/aesthesia." The last part of the word means "feeling or sensibility" and is actually a root word.

Rule Number Six

The use of more than one root word in a medical term creates the need for combining vowels to connect the different roots. This, in turn, creates combining forms used in compound words. In the word "cholangiopancreatography," there are three root words strung together. In the case of "chol" and "angi," there is no need for a combining vowel because the second word already starts with a vowel. In the case, of "angi" and "pancreat," however, the second root word starts with a consonant, so the letter "o" is used between the two root words.

A clearer example appears when the first root word ends with a consonant and the second root word starts with a consonant. Rarely would these two types of words be put together without a combining vowel. Take the example of "megalomaniac,"which means "one who has delusions of grandeur." The word is divided like this: "megal/o/mania/c." The "o" is necessary to make the word easier to say out loud.

Rule Number Seven

To define a medical word, you generally start with trying to understand the suffix (the word ending) first and then continue to"read"backward through the word. This is basically what we've done when defining a word. We start with the suffix to get a sense of what the word is about, and then we back up to see the root word. This is basically done when there is no prefix to look at. (See the next rule.)

Let's look at a couple of simple medical terms:

- **Blepharitis:** this breaks into "blephar/itis" or "inflammation of the eyelid." The suffix defines it as an inflammation of something, while the root word identifies the eyelid as being inflamed.

- **Otalgia:** this breaks into "ot/algia" or "ear pain." Again, the suffix defines the word as being related to pain, and the root word identifies the ear as being painful.

- **Audiology:** this breaks up into "audi/ology" or the "study of the ear." The suffix tells you it is the study of something, and the root word says it's the ear that is being studied.

- **Melanoma:** this divides into "melan/oma." The suffix means it is a type of tumor, and the root word, backing up, says it's a "black tumor," which is the most common color of this type of skin cancer.

- **Somniphobia:** this is divided into "somn/i/phobia" or "the fear of sleep." The suffix "phobia" is a common one used to describe the fear of something. There is the root word meaning sleep, plus the combining vowel "i".

Rule Number Eight

When a medical word has a prefix, you need to define the suffix first, the prefix second, and the root(s) last. You already know this when it comes to defining, but it also applies to building a potential medical term. Think about what the broad category is, which will help you know the suffix to choose. Suffix definitions usually link back to just one particular suffix (as opposed to prefixes, which can have more than one prefix that match the same meaning).

The only exception rule to this is that there is more than one suffix that means "of or pertaining to." The suffixes "ia," "y," and "al" all mean "of or pertaining to." Some suffixes have been anglicized so they have separate Greek, Latin, or English suffixes that mean the same thing. Look at "genesis" and "geny." These both mean generation or origin. The first suffix is Greek and the second is English. So we have:

- Pathogenesis (disease origin) and not "pathogeny," which essentially means the same thing.

- Progeny (one's children) and not "progenesis" or "progeneses" (the plural form of "progenesis").

Prefixes, as mentioned, are more difficult. Do you use "ecto" or "exo"? The word "exogenous" or "originating outside of something" means the same as "ectogenous," but the latter word isn't a real word. In the same way, "ectoplasm" is not "exoplasm," although they could mean the same thing.

Fortunately, most root words have a single meaning and vice versa. These are the last word parts you look at in order to build a word. Many words, real and not real, can be created with root words. Take the suffix "ectomy" or the "removal of something" and put any medical root word in front of it and you can make a case for that word being real. This includes words like these:

- Dermectomy—not a real word, meaning removal of the skin
- Pancreatectomy—a real word, meaning removal of the pancreas
- Gastrectomy—a real word, meaning removal of the stomach
- Sinusectomy—not a real word, meaning removal of the sinuses

See how it's not that easy to build a medical word from scratch without getting away from normal medical conventions?

Rule Number Nine

When a medical word relates to body systems or parts, unveiling the word's meaning usually starts with defining the suffix first, then defining the organs in the order in which they are studied in the body system being studied. "Cholangiopancreatography" is listed as such because the biliary tree is studied before the pancreas. This is why the term "pancreatocholangiogram" is not a word. Fortunately, there are not too many commonly-used medical terms that string two root words together.

Of course, some of it makes no sense at all. What about the term "renovascular hypertension"? The word "renovascular" is constructed as "ren/o/vascul/ar," which strings together the root words for "kidney" and "blood vessel" respectively. It could go either way; however, "vasculorenal" isn't a word. (But technically, it could be, because there is nothing in the rule saying one root word belongs before the other.) This is where convention comes in. You'll find examples throughout medical terminology, where convention has dictated what the word ultimately looks like after it is built.

CHAPTER 3:

TYPES OF PREFIXES

We've seen a lot of prefixes so far, but there are certain prefix types worth looking at further. In this chapter, we will talk about prefix linking to root words, prefixes of number, prefixes of direction, and prefixes of position. Some prefixes you've already learned, but they have a specific role in medical terminology that make them worth mentioning again.

Prefix Linking

There are no specific rules about whether or not to use a hyphen when writing a word with a prefix. Some words naturally link with a hyphen, while others link as a single word. When in doubt, try the word without a prefix as, in medical terminology, there are few hyphens. Medical professionals like to string words into one long word without using hyphens, if at all possible.

Here are some prefixes and the root words they might be linked to. Unlike the links between root words and suffixes, there are no combining vowels between prefixes and the root word. For example, the word "pancytopenia" is not "panocytopenia." It is fully acceptable to combine prefixes that end with a consonant along with root words that begin with a consonant. Let's practice:

- **Anti-.** This means "against or opposed to." In medicine, "anti-reflux" medications are used to prevent reflux (heartburn). This is an example where a hyphen is necessary. "Anti-inflammatory" medications are those against inflammation. There are also "antibiotics," which is a word that does not need a hyphen.

- **Auto-.** This means "self" and helps build words like "autoimmune" diseases, which involve self-antibodies. The word "autophagy" means "consumption of the body's own tissue as a metabolic process occurring in starvation."

- **De-**. This means to reverse or change. "Decontamination" involves reversing contamination, while "deactivate" involves reversing the activation of something.

- **Dis-**. This involves reversing or removing something. "Disease" is the "removal of ease," or a medical disorder. "Disorder" is the removal of "order."

- **Extra-**. This means "beyond." An "extranodal metastasis" is a cancer that has spread beyond the lymph nodes.

- **Hyper-**. This can mean "extreme" and is used in medical terms like "hypertension" (high blood pressure), "hyperextension" (over-extension of the joint), and "hyperacusis" (extreme sensitivity to noise).

- **Inter-**. This means "between." In medicine, "intercellular junctions" are junctions between the cells.

- **Mega-**. This means "very big or important." In nonmedical terms, there is "mega-deal," which is hyphenated. But in medicine, terms like "toxic megacolon" are not hyphenated; this term means "a very large, distended colon." "Megalomania," or "extreme delusions of grandeur," also does not have a hyphen.

- **Mid-**. This means "middle." In medicine, "midabdominal" pain is located in the middle of the abdomen.

- **Mis-**. This means "incorrectly or badly." A "misaligned" fracture is badly aligned. A "miscarriage" is a badly carried pregnancy.

- **Non-**. This means "not." The term "nonsense mutation" is a DNA mutation that does not code for anything because the codons do not make sense.

- **Over-**. This means "too much." In medicine, an "overactive bladder" is one that is too active.

- **Post-**. This means "after." Words like "postoperative," "posterior," and "posthumous.".

- **Pre-**. This means "before." This prefix goes into "prenatal" and "preverbal"—both of which are medical terms. The word "prewar" and "pre-war" can be used with or without a hyphen and are not medical terms.

- **Pro-**. This means "in favor of." The term "prophylactic" does not require a hyphen, while "prodemocracy" and "pro-democracy" can be used either way. In medical terms, try to avoid the hyphen unless it is necessary by convention.

- **Semi-**. This means "half." The "semilunar valves" are valves with leaflets that are in a half-moon shape.

- **Trans-**. This means "across." A "transatlantic flight" goes across the Atlantic Ocean, and the "transphenoidal approach" is a surgical technique that involves going across the sphenoidal sinus. Note the loss of the "s" in between the prefix and root word.

Types of Prefixes

There are many types of prefixes, which basically refer to prefixes that have the same (or similar) meanings. There are, for example **prefixes of negation**. What are some of these prefixes? Let's look:

- Un—as in undesirable, unhappy, unrepentant, undecided, etc.
- Mis—as in misguided, misdirected, mistake, misspelled, misinterpret, etc.
- De—as in demerit, deactivation, deforestation, decapitation, dethrone, etc.
- Mal—as in maltreatment, malfunction, malrotation, malnutrition, maladjustment, etc.
- Non—as in nonsense, nonreactive, nonentity, nondescript, etc.
- Ab—as in abnormal, abduction, etc.
- In—as in insufficient, inability, insensitive, inorganic, inoperable, etc.
- Pseudo—as in pseudocyst, pseudopod, pseudocyesis, etc.

It should be noted that the prefix "in" becomes "im" when it comes before a root word beginning with "b," "p," or "m." This leads to words like immobile, impatient, imbalance, and immature. This is simply a spelling change in the prefix "im," not a new prefix. It is still a negation prefix. "In" can also become "ir" or "il" in words that have root words starting with these letters. For example, there is "illogical," "illegal," "irresponsible," "irresistible," etc.

There are **prefixes of attitude** that indicate being for, with, or against something. For example, here are some prefixes of attitude:

- Anti—this means "against" and includes antipathy, antisocial, antifreeze, etc.
- Pro—this means "for" and includes pronoun, proactive, promotion, prodromal, etc.
- Co—this means "with" and includes codependent, coincidence, coordinate, cooperate, etc.
- Counter—this means "against" and includes counterattack, counterclockwise, countermove, etc.
- Contra—this means "against" and includes contraceptive, contraindication, contralateral, etc.

There are many **prefixes referring to number**, which will be shown later in this chapter. The basic ones are uni, bi/di, tri, quad, tetra, pent, quint, deca, noni, sext, deci, and multi. You'll find that there is more than one prefix that means the same thing when it comes to number prefixes.

Prefixes emphasizing degree are also appropriate in medical terminology. These represent too much, too little, too big, or too small. Some of these include the following:

- Super—this means "big" and includes supersonic, supermarket, supernormal, etc.
- Mini—this means "very small" and includes minibus, miniskirt, miniscule, etc.
- Hyper—this means "too much" and includes hyperventilate, hyperinflated, hypersensitive, etc.
- Over—this means "too much" and includes oversized, overinflated, oversimplify, etc.
- Out—this means "much or more" and includes outwitted, outsmarted, outspoken, etc.

There are many prefixes referred to as **additive or diminutive prefixes.** These are usually a matched set that will indicate words opposite to one another. Some examples include the following:

- Appreciate versus depreciate
- Accelerate versus decelerate

- Absent versus present

- Decrease versus increase

- Displace versus replace

- Deflate versus inflate

- Explode versus implode

- Emigrate versus immigrate

- Export versus import

- Inflow versus outflow

You've already learned the many **prefixes of color**. There are also several prefixes that indicate the **location or direction** of something. Some of these include "pre," which means before in order, position, rank, or time. Words like this include prenatal, predate, prefrontal, prefix, etc. The opposite prefix to this is "post," which means after. Posthumous, postnatal, postoperative, and postdoctoral are words that can be understood in this context. In the same way, there is "trans," which means across or beyond. This prefix combines to become transcutaneous, transverse, and transcendental, among others.

Prefixes of Position

Prefixes of position are commonly used in medicine to describe the position of something in relation to something else in the body. These provide a way of relating two things in the body in space, or identifying the location of something in the body. Let's look at some prefixes that are considered prefixes of position:

- **Epi.** This means "above or upon."

- **Hypo.** This means "under, below, or deficient in something."

- **Infra.** This means "under or below."

- **Sub.** This also means "under or below."

- **Inter.** This means "between."

- **Intra.** This means "within."

- **Post.** This means "after or behind."

- **Pre.** This means "before or in front of."

- **Pro.** This also means "before or in front of."
- **Retro.** This means "backward or behind."
- **Supra.** This means "above."

Using Prefixes of Position in Medicine

Because a great many medical terms relate to position in the body, the prefixes of position are used quite often. Once you know the different prefixes, things like muscles, nerves, and blood vessels, in particular, are easily positioned by the prefixes used to identify them. Let's look at some medical terms that make use of these common prefixes:

- **Epi.** Episcleritis is "epi/scler/it is" or inflammation of an area overlying the sclera. Epigastric is "epi/gastr/ic" or pertaining to something above the stomach.
- **Hypo.** Hypodermic is "hypo/derm/ic" or pertaining to something under the skin. The hypogastric artery ("hypo/gastr/ic") is obviously located beneath the stomach.
- **Infra.** The infrapatellar ligament ("infra/patell/ar") is located beneath the patella or kneecap. The infraorbital area ("infra/orbit/al") is located beneath the orbit or the eye.
- **Sub.** The subcostal ("sub/cost/al") muscles and subcostal nerve are located beneath the ribs.
- **Inter.** The intercostal muscles ("inter/cost/al") are located between the ribs. The intercellular junctions ("inter/cellul/ar") are between the cells. The interosseus ("inter/osse/us") is between two bones.
- **Intra.** The intracellular space ("intra/cellul/ar") is located within the cells themselves. The intraluminal pressure ("intra/lumin/al") is the pressure within the lumen of the GI tract.
- **Post.** The postnatal period ("post/nat/al") is the time period after birth. The postpartum period ("post/partum") is similar, but refers to the time period after pregnancy.
- **Pre.** The prenatal visit ("pre/nat/al") is a visit performed during pregnancy. The preconception period ("pre/concept/ion") is the time period before a baby is

conceived.

- **Pro.** To procreate ("pro/create") refers to "before creation," as in to start a family.

- **Retro.** A retroverted ("retro/vert/ed") uterus is one that has tilted backward. The retroperitoneal space ("retro/peritone/al") is behind the peritoneal space in the abdomen.

- **Supra.** The supraspinatus muscle ("supra/spinat/us") is located above the spine of the scapula and is above the infraspinatus muscle ("infra/spinat/us"), located below the spine.

Prefixes of Number

Let's look at prefixes that refer to number first and identify medical terms that have these word parts in them:

- **Nulli-.** This prefix means "none" and is used in words such as "nulliparous," which represents someone who has never had a child. The term "nulligravida," on the other hand, refers to never having been pregnant.

- **Haplo-.** This prefix means "single" and is used in words such as "haplotype," which means "half of a type," a word that is often used in genetics to represent half of a chromosome.

- **Mon-, mono-.** These prefixes mean "one" and are used in words such as "monopoly," which means exclusive control of a commodity or service in a particular market. The prefix "mono" refers to a single entity having control. In medicine and botany, it is used in words such as "monospermous," which means having one seed.

- **Bi-, di-, dipl-.** These prefixes mean "two, double or twice" and are used in words such as "biceps," which refers to something that has two heads. For example, the "biceps muscle" has two heads.

- **Tri-.** This prefix means "three" and is used in words such as "triceps," which refers to something that has three heads. For example, the "triceps muscle" has three heads.

- **Tetra-.** This prefix refers to the number "four" and is used in words such as "tetralogy of Fallot," which is a disease of the heart that involves four different cardiac anomalies, first identified by Dr. Fallot. It can also mean a group of four dramas, three tragedies and one satyr play, performed consecutively at the festival of Dionysus in ancient Athens. Another word that can be used with this prefix is "tetragram," which means a word of four letters.

- **Penta-.** This prefix refers to the number "five" and is used in words such as "pentagram." A pentagram is a five-pointed, star-shaped figure made by extending the sides of a regular pentagon until they meet; it was used as an occult symbol by the Pythagoreans and later by philosophers, magicians, and others.

- **Hex-, sex-.** These prefixes refer to the number "six" and are used in words such as "hexagram." A hexagram is a six-pointed star-like figure formed of two equilateral triangles placed concentrically, with each side of a triangle parallel to a side of the other and on opposite sides of the center. In medicine, it is used in words such as "hexapodous," which means having six feet.

- **Octo-, Octa-.** These prefixes refer to the number "eight" and are used in words such as "octopus," which is any octopod of the genus Octopus, having a soft, oval body and eight sucker-bearing arms, living mostly at the bottom of the sea.

- **Nona-.** This prefix refers to the number "nine" and is used in words that refer to having nine of something. This isn't commonly used in medical terminology, but it is used for completeness. It can mean "sleeping sickness."

- **Deci-.** This prefix refers to the number "ten" and is used in words such as "decimeter," which means a unit of length equal to 1/10 (0. 1) meter.

- **Primi/o-.** This prefix refers to the ordinal number "first" and is used in words such as "primiparous," which means a woman who has borne only one child or who is parturient for the first time.

- **Hemi-.** This prefix refers to "half" or "one side" and is used in words such as "hemisphere," which is defined as half of a sphere. In anatomy, it can mean either of the lateral halves of the cerebrum or cerebellum.

- **Semi-.** This prefix refers to "half" or "partial" and is used in words such as "semispherical," which means something that is shaped like half a sphere, hemispheric.

- **Quadr/o-.** This prefix refers to the number "four" and is used in words such as

44

"quadrilateral," which means a plane figure having four sides and four angles.

- **Multi-.** This prefix refers to "many" and is used in words such as "multiple," which means manifold, or consisting of, having, or involving several individuals, parts, elements, relations, etc..

- **Poly-.** This prefix refers to "many" or "much" and is used in words such as "polygamy," which means the habit or system of mating with more than one individual, either simultaneously or successively.

- **Dodeca-.** This prefix means "twelve" and is a prefix referring to that number. It is used in words such as "dodecahedron," which is a solid figure having twelve faces.

- **Proto-.** This prefix refers to the ordinal number "first." It is used as a prefix to define the order of things and is used in words such as "prototype," which means the first of a kind with regard tot an invention.

- **Deuter-.** This prefix refers to the ordinal number "second" and is a prefix used to identify the order of things. A word that uses this prefix is "deuteropathy," which means (in pathology) any abnormality that is secondary to another pathological condition.

- **Tripl-.** This prefix means "triple." It is used in words such as "triploblastic," which means (in zoology) having three primary germ layers, as the embryos of vertebrates.

- **Quadri-.** This prefix means "four" and refers to something having four of something. It is used in words such as "quadriceps," which (in medicine) means a large muscle in front of the thigh, the action of which extends the leg or bends the hip joint.

- **Hepta-.** This prefix means "seven" and refers to something having seven of something. When it is used in a medical term, it means that something consists of (or is divided into) seven parts.

- **Enna(e)-.** This prefix means "nine" and refers to having nine of something. It is used in medical terminology as the word "ennaeaphyllous," which means dividing something or consisting of nine parts.

- **Deca-.** This prefix means "ten" and refers to having ten of something. In medical terms, it is used in the word "decamerous," which means consisting of ten parts or divisions.

- **Hect-**. This prefix means "one hundred" and refers to having a hundred of something. It is used in the word "hectoliter," which means a unit of capacity equal to 100 liters.

- **Kil-**. This prefix means "one thousand" and refers to having a thousand of something. It is used in the word "kilometer," which means a unit of length, the common measure of distances equal to 1000 meters, equivalent to 3280. 8 feet or 0.621 of a mile.

- **Uni-**. This prefix means "one" and refers to having one of something. A word with this prefix is "unicostate," which means having only one costa, rib, or ridge or, in biology (of a leaf), having only one primary or prominent rib (the midrib).

- **Du-**. This prefix means "two" and refers to having two of something. It is used in the word "dual," which means composed or consisting of two people, items, parts, etc..

- **Bin-**. This prefix means "two" and refers to having two of something. In medicine, it is used in the word "binaural," which means of, with, or for both ears. For example, having binaural hearing or a binaural stethoscope. "Binary language" in computers involves only two numbers.

- **Second-**. This prefix means "second" and refers to the order of things. It is used in the term "secondary," meaning that something pertains to the second of two things.

- **Secundi-**. This prefix means "second" and refers to the order of things. It is used in the word "secundigravida," which means being pregnant for the second time.

- **Terti-**. This prefix means "third" and refers to the order of things. It is used in the word "tertiary," which means the third of something.

- **Quadru-**. This prefix means "four" and refers to having four of something. An example of this prefix is in the word "quadrupedal," which means an animal, especially a mammal, having four feet.

- **Quinque-**. This prefix means "five" and refers to having five of something. It is used in the word "quinquilateral," which means an object having five sides. This is closely related to "quint," as in "quintuplets."

- **Sex-.** This prefix means "six" and refers to having six of something. It is used in the word "sextant," which is an astronomical instrument used to determine latitude and longitude at sea.

- **Sept-.** This prefix refers to the number "seven" and refers to having seven of something. It is used in the word "septuple," which means sevenfold, or consisting of seven parts.

- **Noni-.** This prefix refers to the number "nine" and refers to having nine of something. It is used in the word "nonipara," which means being pregnant for the ninth time.

- **Centi-.** This prefix refers to the number "one hundred" and refers to having a hundred of something. It is used in the word "centipede," which means having a hundred legs.

- **Milli-.** This prefix means "one thousand" and refers to having a thousand of something. It is used in the word "millipede," which means having a thousand legs.

Using Prefixes of Number in Medicine

Medicine uses prefixes related to number in all aspects of medicine. Everyone knows the terms used to identify multiple births, from "twins" to "triplets" ("tri/plets") to "octuplets" ("octu/plets") and all numbers of multiples in between. The term "nullipara" and "nulligravida" both mean "none" of something. In the case of nulligravida, it refers to never having been pregnant, while the term nullipara refers to never having given birth. A woman who is nulliparous may or may not be nulligravida (because she might be pregnant but hasn't given birth yet).

Prefixes of Measurement

We've covered some of these already but, when it comes to measurement, these prefixes can mean something slightly different than what we've discussed. Here are common prefixes related to measurement:

- **Centi.** This can refer to a hundred but can also refer to one hundredth of something.

- **Milli.** This can refer to a thousand or to a thousandth of something.

- **Centi, hecto, hect, or hecato.** These refer to a hundred of something in measurement terms.

- **Kilo.** This refers to a thousand of something in measurement terms.

- **Semi or hemi.** These both refer to half of something.

- **Sesqui.** This refers to one-and-a-half of something.

- **Multi or poly.** These refer to many of something.

- **Deci.** This can refer to ten or to a tenth of something.

- **Deca.** This specifically refers to ten of something.

- **Mega.** In measurement terms, this refers to one million of something.

- **Micro.** This refers to one millionth of something.

- **Giga.** This refers to a billion of something

- **Nano.** This refers to a billionth of something.

- **Pico.** This refers to a trillionth of something.

- **Femto.** This refers to a quadrillionth of something.

Using Prefixes of Measurement in Medicine

When it comes to prefixes related to measurement in medicine, it's best to look at how these prefixes play into science and medicine, in general, in common (and some uncommon) measurements. Let's take the liter, the meter, and the gram as examples of common measurements used in scientific and medical circles. These are commonly multiplied or divided to get measurements that are more conveniently expressed. For example:

- Kilogram — this is equal to a thousand grams.

- Kilometer — this is equal to a thousand meters.

- Deciliter — this is one tenth of a liter.

- Milliliter — this is one thousandth of a liter.

- Microliter—this is one millionth of a liter.

- Femtoliter—this is one quadrillionth of a liter.

- Micrometer—this is a millionth of a meter.

- Millimeter—this is one thousandth of a meter.

- Nanogram—this is a billionth of a gram.

- Picogram—this is a trillionth of a gram.

- Gigabyte—this is used in computer terminology to recognize a billion bytes.

The examples listed above are the more commonly used derivations of measurements used in medicine and science. Technically, although decigram isn't commonly used, it can be easily defined as a tenth of a gram. That's why it's so important to identify the prefixes of measurement and to know what they mean.

Prefixes of Direction

Prefixes of direction generally imply action or movement. For example, the act of abduction and adduction of the extremities are important things to know because they mean the opposite of one another—and it is easy to confuse them. When you know the different prefix meanings, however, the actions become clearer. Let's look at some prefixes of direction:

- **Ab.** This means "away from."

- **Ad.** This means "toward."

- **E-.** This means "out or away."

- **Circum.** This means "around."

- **Peri.** This means "around."

- **Pro.** This means "forward."

- **Retro.** This means "backward."

Using Prefixes of Direction in Medicine

As mentioned, prefixes of direction usually imply movement or action. They tend to be used in words that are related to an action or to the movement of something.

- **Ab.** This means "away from." To abduct an extremity means to move it away from the center of the body.

- **Ad.** This means "toward." Adduction, or the act of adducting an extremity, involves bringing it toward the center of the body. The adductor muscles are those muscles that do this action.

- **E-.** This means "out or away." To evoke something is to bring it out. To evaporate something ("e/vapor/ate") means to remove water or take water out.

- **Circum.** This means "around." The term "circumoral" refers to something (a rash or cyanosis) around the mouth.

- **Peri.** This means "around." The perianal area is the skin around the anus. The perinatal period is the period around the time of birth. This prefix is also used to make the word describing the time around menopause (perimenopause).

- **Pro.** This means "forward." The act of pronation is to rotate the shoulders forward or to rotate the hand so that the back of the hand is facing forward. It also means the inward turning of the soles of the feet at the ankle. To proliferate is to grow or multiply quickly.

- **Retro.** This means "backward." Retroversion of the uterus involves a tipping of the uterus in the backward direction. Retroflexion is the flexion of the uterus backward from its normal position (which is usually in the forward position).

So, while you may not know every single prefix possible in medicine, this is an excellent start. Memorize these and you should be well on your way to understanding many different types of medical and nonmedical terms.

CHAPTER 4:

TYPES OF SUFFIXES

Suffixes (the end of a word) are looked at first when defining a term—for a reason. It's because the suffix truly does define and change the meaning of a word. You have learned many suffixes, and you have also learned how they help you know what a word is about. In this chapter, we will take a closer look at suffixes so you can know what the classifications are, as well as what they mean.

Suffix Linking

Suffixes are the word part at the end of the word and may be either singular or plural. While there are few changes to the connection between a prefix and the root word, there are often changes to the root word or the suffix in order to make the word more manageable to say. This, as you know, involves the use of a combining vowel. Most often, the vowel is "o," but it can be "i" or "a" in some cases.

In general, suffixes that begin with a vowel are linked directly to the word root, while suffixes that begin with a consonant are linked using a combining vowel. Sometimes, however, it is hard to know what the suffix actually is. For example, is it "dermat/o/logy" or is it "dermat/ology"? In fact, the answer depends on the Greek or Latin word underlying the suffix. In this case, the suffix stems from the word Greek word "logos," which means "word; reason." It helps to make the suffixes "logy" and "logist," where the latter is the suffix meaning "a specialist in something."

Linking of a suffix using these linking rules happens like this:

- Cardiomegaly—this breaks down into "cardi/o/megaly." In such cases, the suffix starts with a consonant, so there is a combining vowel used.

- Cardiac—this breaks down into "cardi/ac." The root word is "heart" and the suffix "ac" means "pertaining to." This starts with a vowel, so there is no need to have a combining vowel form between the two different word parts.

Three Main Categories of Suffixes

In medical terminology, suffixes are unique in that there are certain types that mean certain things. When you know the different suffixes under the different categories, you will know broadly what these terms mean. The three main categories in the medical terminology of suffixes include surgical suffixes, diagnostic/pathological suffixes, and grammatical suffixes. You'll see grammatical suffixes in everyday language; however, the surgical and diagnostic/pathological suffixes tend to be unique in medicine so, when these are seen, you can be relatively assured that the term is a medical one.

Surgical Suffixes

Surgical suffixes are used to define a surgical procedure, or related procedure, in medicine. These should be memorized as they give a wealth of information as to exactly what is being done as part of the procedure. As always, they are connected to root words that round out the meaning of the word and give you a complete picture of what the term really means.

These are the terms you should memorize:

- **Centesis.** This means "to puncture a cavity to remove fluid." It is used in the word "amniocentesis," which is a procedure in which fluid is removed from the amniotic sac for evaluation.

- **Ectomy.** This means "to excise or surgically remove." It is used in many terms, "hysterectomy" being one of them. The term refers to the surgical removal of the uterus.

- **Ostomy.** This involves "a new permanent opening." A tracheostomy is a permanent hole in the trachea.

- **Otomy.** This means "incision" or "cutting into." A gastrotomy means to cut into the stomach surgically.

- **Orrhaphy.** This means "surgical repair or suture." A "herniorrhaphy" is the surgical repair of a swelling or hernia.

- **Opexy.** This means "surgical fixation." For example, in a "nephropexy," the kidney is fixated to the abdominal wall.

- **Oplasty.** This simply means "surgical repair." In a "rhinoplasty," the nose is surgically repaired.

- **Otripsy.** This means "to crush or destroy." It can be used to make "lithotripsy," which is the crushing of stones in the urinary tract.

Using Surgical Suffixes

These eight surgical suffixes comprise the vast majority of surgical procedures that are used in medicine. There are many ways to use these suffixes when creating or identifying medical terms:

- **Centesis.** Let's look at this suffix, which involves "removing fluid." The term "paracentesis" is divided into "para/centesis," which involves the removal of abdominal fluid, either for evaluation or for therapeutic purposes. An "arthrocentesis," or "arthr/o/centesis," means the removal of the fluid in a joint for analysis or therapeutic reasons. A "pericardiocentesis," or "peri/cardi/o/centesis," is the removal of fluid from the pericardial sac around the heart.

- **Ectomy.** This means "to excise or surgically remove." This is probably used the most in surgical words. There is "gastrectomy," "pancreatectomy," and "colectomy," which mean the removal of the stomach, pancreas, and colon, respectively. Just about any body area can be translated into "the removal of" by adding -ectomy to the end of the medical root word.

- **Ostomy.** This means to create "a new permanent opening." An "iliostomy," which is divided into "ili/ostomy," means to create a permanent opening in the ilium. In the same way, "jejunostomy" (or "jejun/ostomy") means to create a permanent opening into the jejunum. A "colostomy" is a common term that means to create a permanent hole in the colon that opens to the outside.

- **Otomy.** This means "incision" or "cutting into" and is another common medical term. A "phlebotomy" (or "phleb/otomy") means to take blood by cutting into or puncturing a vein. A "tracheotomy" (or "trache/otomy") is the process of cutting into the trachea. It doesn't necessarily mean that the hole created is permanent.

- **Orrhaphy.** This means "surgical repair or suture." A "gastrorrhaphy" (or "gastr/orrhaphy") is the surgical repair of the stomach. There is more than one word that means "surgical repair," so it may be difficult to actually build a word without paying attention to medical convention.

- **Opexy.** This means "surgical fixation" and implies affixing a body part that is not in its correct place. An example is "orchiopexy" (or "orchi/opexy"), which means the surgical fixation of the testicles or testes when they are not in their correct position. A "mastopexy" involves the fixation or lifting of the breast or "a breast lift."

- **Oplasty.** This simply means "surgical repair." This is commonly used in plastic surgery procedures and includes "blepharoplasty" (or "blephar/oplasty"), which means the surgical repair of the eyelid in plastic surgery. "Otoplasty" (or "ot/oplasty") means to surgically repair the ear.

- **Otripsy.** This means "to crush or destroy." This is not commonly used in medicine and is sometimes referred to as "tripsy" without the "o." A "cephalotripsy" (or "cephal/otripsy") is the crushing of the skull.

Diagnostic, Pathological, and Related Suffixes

These are terms that mainly refer to something medical, so you won't see them used in nonmedical circles. Though there are more of them out there, these bear memorizing because they will help you understand the core meaning of the word. Let's take a look at these suffixes:

- **Algia.** This means "pain" and is used in words like "myalgia," which means muscle pain.

- **Emia.** This means "blood" and is used in words like "hypoglycemia," which means low blood sugar.

- **Itis.** This means "inflammation" and is used in terms like "bronchitis," which means bronchial tube inflammation.

- **Lysis.** This means "destruction or breakdown" and is used in "autolysis," which means the destruction of the self.

- **Oid.** This means "like" and is used to make "diploid," which means double or like two.

- **Opathy.** This means "disease of" and is used in "arthropathy," or disease of the joints.

- **Pnea.** This means "breathing" and is used in "apnea," which means not breathing.

- **Dynia.** This means "pain" and is used in "allodynia," which means pain all over.

- **Cele.** This means "hernia or swelling" and is used in "rectocele," which is a swelling/hernia of the rectum.

- **Ectasis.** This means "expansion or dilation" and is used in "bronchiectasis," which is a dilation of the bronchial tree.

- **Edema.** This means "swelling" and is used in "lymphedema," which is a swelling of the lymph fluid.

- **Emesis.** This means "vomiting" and is used in "hematemesis," which means vomiting of blood.

- **Iasis.** This means "abnormal condition" and is used in "helminthiasis," which is a worm infestation.

- **Lith.** This means "stone" and is used in "ureterolith," which means stone in the ureter.

- **Malacia.** These mean "softening" and is used in "osteomalacia," or bone softening.

- **Oma.** This means "tumor" and is used in "melanoma," which is a type of skin tumor.

- **Osis.** This means "abnormal condition or increase" and is used in "psychosis," which is an abnormal psychiatric condition.

- **Penia.** This means "decrease or deficiency" and is used in "osteopenia," or bone deficiency.

- **Phobia.** This means "fear" and is used in "photophobia," which is a fear of light.

- **Plegia.** This means "paralysis" and is used in "hemiplegia," which is a paralysis of half of the body.

- **Rrhage or Rrhagia.** This means "bursting forth" and is used in "hemorrhage," which means bleeding.

- **Rrhea.** This means "discharge or flow" and is used in "diarrhea," which means loose stools.

- **Rrhexis.** This means "rupture" and is used in "cardiorrhexis," which is a rupture of the heart.

- **Toxic.** This means "poison" and is used in "nephrotoxic," which means poisonous to the kidneys.

- **Trophy.** This means "nourishment or development" and is used in "atrophy," which means a lack of development.

Using Diagnostic, Pathological and Related Suffixes

- **Algia.** This means "pain." The word "arthralgia" (or "arthr/algia") means joint pain, and "otalgia" (or "ot/algia") means ear pain. A synonym for this is "dynia."

- **Emia.** This means "blood." It creates words like "polycythemia" (or "poly/cyt/h/emia"), which is a condition of too many cells in the blood. The word "uremia" (or "ur/emia") involves products of the kidneys in the bloodstream.

- **Itis.** This means "inflammation." There are many words used in this context, such as "appendicitis" (or "appendic/i" is"), which is an inflammation of the appendix. Other words, like "myocarditis," "tonsillitis," and "cervicitis" refer to specific areas of inflammation.

- **Lysis.** This means "destruction or break down." The term "hemolysis" (or "hemo/lysis") refers to the breakdown or destruction of blood.

- **Oid.** This means "like." There are several medical words with this suffix, including "haploid" (or "hap/loid"), which refers to half of something. "Chancroid" is like a chancre.

- **Opathy.** This means "disease of." This is commonly used in medicine in terms like "neuropathy" (or "neur/opathy"), which means nerve disease, and "uropathy" (or "ur/opathy"), which means urine disease.

- **Pnea.** This means "breathing." The term "hypopnea" (or "hypo/pnea"), which refers to under-breathing, makes use of this suffix.

- **Dynia.** This means "pain." The medical term "pleurodynia" (or "pleuro/dynia") means lung pain or pain involving the pleural lining.

- **Cele.** This means "hernia or swelling." The medical term "omphalocele" (or "omphalo/cele") refers to a swelling of the abdominal wall from a hernia of the wall at birth. A "cystocele" (or "cysto/cele") is a hernia of the bladder.

- **Ectasis.** This means "expansion or dilation." "Bronchiectasis" (or "bronchi/ectasis") often refers to a dilation of a tubular or hollow organ.

- **Edema.** This means "swelling." The term "angioedema" (or "angio/edema") refers to a swelling of blood vessels.

- **Emesis.** This means "vomiting." The suffix itself is also a medical term, meaning "vomiting."

- **Iasis.** This means "abnormal condition." The term "hypochondriasis" (or "hypo/chondr/iasis") doesn't mean anything close to what it sounds like it should mean. It refers to a morbid concern about one's health.

- **Lith.** This means "stone." It is not used in many medical terms. The term "fecalith" (or "feca/lith") means hard feces or a "fecal stone."

- **Malacia.** These means "softening." It is often used in orthopedics. For example, "chondromalacia" (or "chondro/malacia") means a softening of the cartilage.

- **Oma.** This means "tumor." An "osteoma" (or "oste/oma") is a bone tumor, while a "chondroma" is a cartilage tumor.

- **Osis.** This means "abnormal condition or increase." The term "leukocytosis" (or "leuko/cyt/osis") means an abnormal increase or elevation in the count of white blood cells.

- **Penia.** This means "decrease or deficiency." This is used in several terms, such as "leukopenia" (or "leuko/penia"), which is a deficiency or decrease in white blood cells.

- **Phobia.** This means "fear." There are many "phobias" in medical terminology. The term of "arachnophobia" (or "arachno/phobia") means a fear of spiders. "Claustrophobia" (or "claustr/o/phobia") is a fear of enclosed spaces.

- **Plegia.** This means "paralysis." "Paraplegia" (or "para/plegia") is a paralysis of the legs, while "quadriplegia" (or "quadr/i/plegia") is a paralysis of all four limbs in a human.

- **Rrhage or Rrhagia.** This means "bursting forth." The term "menorrhagia" (or "men/o/rrhagia") is heavy menstrual flow.

- **Rrhea.** This means "discharge or flow." The medical term "hypermenorrhea" (or "hyper/men/o/rrhea") is an excess of menstrual bleeding. "Rhinorrhea" (or "rhino/rrhea") is a runny nose.

- **Rrhexis.** This means "rupture." There are actually several terms used in medicine that make use of this suffix, but they aren't common. "Phleborrhexis" (or "phlebo/rrhexis") is the rupture of a vein, while "tubulorrhexis" (or "tubul/o/rrhexis") is the rupture of a tube.

- **Toxic.** This means "poison." The term "hemotoxic" (or "hemo/toxic") means poisonous to the blood. The complex word "thyrotoxicosis" (or "thyr/o/toxic/osis") is a term meaning an excessive poisoning of the thyroid hormone.

- **Trophy.** This means "nourishment or development." The term "hypertrophy" (or "hyper/trophy") means excessive development.

Grammatical Suffixes

These can be suffixes used in everyday language, but they definitely have a place in medical terminology. There are three types of grammatical suffixes: those that refer to nouns, those that refer to adjectives, and those that indicate the diminutive of something. Let's take a look at some common grammatical suffixes in medical terms:

- **Ac.** This indicates an adjective and means "pertaining to," as in the word "cardiac," which means pertaining to the heart.

- **Al.** This is an adjective suffix meaning "pertaining to." It is seen in the word "neural," which means pertaining to the nerves.

- **Ar.** This is an adjective suffix meaning "pertaining to." It is used in "muscular," which means pertaining to muscle.

- **Ary.** This is an adjective suffix meaning "pertaining to." It is used in "pulmonary," which means pertaining to the lungs.

- **Eal.** This is an adjective suffix meaning "pertaining to" and is seen in "esophageal," which means pertaining to the esophagus.

- **Ic.** This is an adjective suffix meaning "pertaining to" and is seen in "thoracic," which means pertaining to the chest.

- **Ical.** This is an adjective suffix meaning "pertaining to" and is seen in "logical," which means pertaining to reason or word (see "logos" above).

- **Ile.** This is an adjective suffix meaning "pertaining to" and is seen in "penile," which means pertaining to the penis.

- **Ior.** This is an adjective suffix meaning "pertaining to." It is seen in "posterior," which means pertaining to the back.

- **Ous.** This is an adjective suffix meaning "pertaining to." It is used in "cutaneous," which means pertaining to the skin.

- **Tic.** This is an adjective suffix meaning "pertaining to." It is used in "acoustic," which means pertaining to hearing.

- **Esis.** This is a noun suffix meaning "condition." It is used in "diuresis," which means a condition of fluid loss through the kidneys.

- **Ia.** This is a noun suffix meaning "condition." It is used in "pneumonia," which means a condition of the lungs.

- **Ism.** This is a noun suffix meaning "condition." It is used in "hypothyroidism," which means a low thyroid condition.

- **Iatry.** This is a noun suffix meaning "medicine or treatment." It is used in "podiatry," which means foot medicine.

- **Ician.** This is a noun suffix meaning "specialist." It is used in "musician," which means a specialist in music.

- **Ist.** This is a noun suffix meaning "specialist." It is used in "podiatrist," which means a specialist in foot medicine.

- **Y.** This is a noun suffix meaning "condition or process," as in "trisomy," which means three bodies.

- **Icle.** This is a diminutive suffix meaning "small or minute," as in "ventricle" — a chamber of the heart.

- **Ole.** This is a diminutive suffix meaning "small or minute," as in "arteriole," which means a small artery.
- **Ule.** This is a diminutive suffix meaning "small or minute," as in "venule," which means a small vein.

Using Grammatical Suffixes

As you have seen, there are many suffixes meaning "pertaining to" and "condition," as well as those which are diminutive in nature, meaning "small." This provides a wealth of choices of suffix endings for a variety of medical terms. A few of these are as follows:

- **Ac.** This means "pertaining to." The term "sciatic" (or "sciat/ic") means pertaining to the lower back (from the Latin "sciaticus"). The term "sacroiliac" (or "sacr/o/ili/ac") means pertaining to the sacrum and ilium.
- **Al.** This means "pertaining to." The term "abdominal" (or "abdomin/al") means pertaining to the abdomen. The term "atrial" (or "atri/al") means pertaining to the atrium of the heart.
- **Ar.** This means "pertaining to." The term "tubular" (or "tubul/ar") means pertaining to a tubule. The term "vascular" (or "vascul/ar") means pertaining to a blood vessel.
- **Ary.** This means "pertaining to." The term "secondary" (or "second/ary") means pertaining to the second of something. The term "coronary" (or "coron/ary") means pertaining to the heart.
- **Eal.** This means "pertaining to." The term "corporeal" (or "corpor/eal") means pertaining to the body. The term "esophageal" (or "esophag/eal") means pertaining to the esophagus.
- **Ic.** This means "pertaining to." The term "aortic" (or "aort/ic") means pertaining to the aorta, while "lipoic" (or "lipo/ic") means pertaining to fat.
- **Ical.** This means "pertaining to." The term "lumbrical" (or "lumbr/ical") means pertaining to a worm (indicating the shape of the lumbrical muscles). The term "optical" (or "opt/ical") means pertaining to the eye.
- **Ile.** This means "pertaining to." The term "senile" (or "sen/ile") means pertaining to diseases of old age (from the Latin "senilis"). The term "infantile" (or

"infant/ile") means pertaining to infancy.

- **Ior.** This means "pertaining to." The term "superior" (or "super/ior") means upper, or pertaining to something above something else. The term "inferior" (or "infer/ior") means pertaining to something below something else.

- **Ous.** This is means "pertaining to." The term "mucous" (or "muc/ous") means pertaining to mucus. The term "vacuous" (or "vacu/ous") means full of air, or pertaining to air.

- **Tic.** This means "pertaining to." The term "optic" (or "op/tic") means pertaining to the eye. The term "therapeutic" (or "therapeu/tic") means pertaining to therapy.

- **Esis.** This means "condition." The term "pseudocyesis" (or "pseudo/cy/esis") means false pregnancy. The term "enuresis" (or "en/ur/esis") refers to a condition of urination.

- **Ia.** This means "condition." The term "alogia" (or "a/log/ia") means a lack of words. The term "myopia" (or "my/op/ia") is a condition of nearsightedness.

- **Ism.** This means "condition." The term "voyeurism" (or "voyeur/ism") means the condition of being a voyeur. The term "neuroticism" (or "neuro/tic/ism") means a condition relating to the nerves.

- **Iatry.** This means "medicine or treatment." The term "psychiatry" (or "psych/iatry") means the treatment of the psyche. The term "physiatry" (or "phys/iatry") means physical medicine.

- **Ician.** This means "specialist." The term "physician" (or "phys/ician") refers to a specialist in physical medicine. The term "beautician" (or beaut/ician) refers to a specialist in beauty.

- **Ist.** This means "specialist." The term "optometrist" (or "opto/metr/ist") refers to a specialist of the eye. The term "physiatrist" (or "phys/iatr/ist") refers to a specialist in physical medicine.

- **Y.** This means "condition or process." The term "primary" (or "primar/y") is a condition or process relating to the first of something. This is related to the term "primarius," which is a Classical Latin term.

- **Icle.** This means "small or minute." The term "auricle" (or "aur/icle") means the earlobe. The "clavicle" (or "clav/icle") is a small bone in the upper chest. It is from the Latin word "clavicula" (or "small key"), which is a diminutive of clavis (because of its shape).

- **Ole.** This means "small or minute." The term "bronchiole" (or "bronchi/ole") means a small bronchus. The term "vacuole" (or "vacu/ole") means a small air-filled organelle in the cell.

- **Ule.** This means "small or minute." The term "tubule" (or "tub/ule") means a small tube. The term "venule" (or "ven/ule") means a small vein.

Now that you're clear on the many prefixes and suffixes in medical terminology, we'll look at specific body areas and the common medical terms you'll come into contact with.

CHAPTER 5:

THE REPRODUCTIVE SYSTEM

In this chapter, we'll first study the root words that apply directly to the reproductive system. These root words usually have to be memorized, although they will be familiar to some. After this, we'll use some of these root words, dissect them, and determine what they mean in practical terms.

Root Words in the Reproductive System

As usual, most of these terms come from the Greek or Latin language and don't always make a great deal of sense. They were created when the study of anatomy and medicine was based on these languages. Memorize these root words and you will unlock a great deal of understanding about the reproductive system:

- **Amni/o.** This refers mainly to the amnion, which is the sac surrounding the embryo.

- **Andr/o.** This is the root term meaning male and is used when things related to the male are referred to.

- **Balan/o.** This is the root word for glans penis.

- **Barthin/o.** This is the root word referring to the Bartholin glands.

- **Blastoma.** This is a suffix word that means immature tumor cells.

- **Cervic/o.** This is the root word for neck or cervix (which is the neck of the uterus).

- **Chori/o or chorion/o.** These are root words meaning chorion, or the outermost membrane covering the fetus.

- **Colp/o.** This is the root word meaning vagina.

- **Culd/o.** This is the root word meaning cul-de-sac.
- **Cyesis.** This is the suffix term for pregnancy.
- **Embry/o.** This is the root word for embryo.
- **Estr/o.** This is the root word used to describe something female.
- **Epididym/o.** This is the root word describing the epididymis.
- **Episi/o.** This is the root term for vulva.
- **Fet/o.** This is the root word referring to fetus.
- **Galact/o.** This is the root word meaning milk.
- **Gest/o.** This is one of the root words describing pregnancy.
- **Gester/o.** This is another root word describing pregnancy.
- **Genit/o.** This is the root word behind those things related to reproduction.
- **Gon/o.** This is the root word for seed.
- **Gonad/o.** This is the root word meaning the sex glands.
- **Gravid/o.** This is a root word related to pregnancy.
- **-Gravida.** This is a suffix meaning a pregnant woman.
- **Gynec/o.** This is the root word used to describe something related to a woman or female.
- **Hymen/o.** This is the root word or phrase related to the female hymen.
- **Hystero.** This is the root word for uterus or womb.
- **Kary/o.** This is the root word for nucleus of the cell.
- **Labi/o.** This is the root word for lip.
- **Lact/o.** This is one of the root words for milk.
- **Lei/o.** This is a root word meaning smooth.
- **Mamm/o.** This is the root word behind "breast."
- **Men/o.** This is the root word for menses or menstruation.
- **Metr/o.** This is a root word for uterus or womb.
- **Metri/o.** This is another root word for uterus or womb.
- **Nat/i.** This is a root word that means "birth."

- **Obstetr/o.** This is a root word meaning birth or pregnancy.
- **Oophoro.** This is the root word meaning ovary.
- **Orch/o.** This is a root word meaning testes.
- **Orchi/o.** This is a root word meaning testes.
- **Orchid/o.** This is another root word meaning testes.
- **Oscheo.** This is a root word meaning scrotum.
- **Ov/o.** This is a root word meaning egg.
- **Ovari/o.** This is a root word meaning ovary.
- **Ovul/o.** This is a root word that means egg.
- **Para.** This refers to bearing or bringing forth, as in the number of live births.
- **Parous.** This is a suffix term meaning to bear or to bring forth.
- **Pareunia.** This is the medical term for sexual intercourse.
- **Partum.** This is the suffix term meaning labor or birth.
- **Perine/o.** This is the root word that means perineum.
- **Phall/o.** This is the root word for the male penis.
- **Prostat/o.** This is the root word that means the male prostate gland.
- **Salpinx.** This is a suffix word referring to the Fallopian tube.
- **Salping/o.** This is the root word for Fallopian tube.
- **Semen/i.** This is the root word for "semen."
- **Sperm/o.** This is a root word for spermatozoa or sperm cells.
- **Spermat/o.** This is another root word for sperm cells or spermatozoa.
- **Terat/o.** This is a root word meaning "monster" or, more clearly, malformed fetus.
- **Test/o.** This is the root word for testis.
- **The/o.** This is the root word for nipple or breast.
- **Toc/o.** This is a root word meaning birth or labor.
- **Tocia.** This is a root word or suffix for a condition of birth or labor.
- **Tocin.** This is a suffix word meaning a substance for birth or labor.
- **Tub/o.** This refers to tube, such as the fallopian tube.

- **Uter/o.** This is a root word for uterus or womb.

- **Vagin/o.** This is a root word pertaining to the vagina.

- **Vesicul/o.** This is a root word for seminal vesicle.

- **Vulv/o.** This is a root word that refers to the female vulva.

Putting it All Together

There are a great many root words, prefixes, and suffixes that relate directly to the reproductive system (of both males and females). With some of these, it's easy to see how they relate to their meaning; others simply have to be memorized. The following are these words used in relationship with real-life terms utilized in medical terminology. They make use of the root words, combined with commonly-used prefixes and suffixes, to create some meaningful words.

Here are some medical terms to remember:

- **Chorioamnionitis.** This divides into "chorio/amnio/n/it/is." It involves an inflammation of the amnion and chorion, which are tissues around the fetus. The medical root word "amnio" means the sac surrounding the embryo, while "chorio" means the outermost layer/membrane around the fetus.

- **Andrology.** This divides into "andr/ology." This is the study of the male reproductive system. It relies on the term "andr," which means male, and "ology," which means the study of.

- **Balanitis.** This refers to the glans penis and is an inflammation of the glans. The root word is "balan," which means glans penis, while "itis" refers to inflammation.

- **Cervical cancer.** This involves cancer of the neck of the "cervix." The root word "cervic" means neck or cervix.

- **Culdocentesis.** This is the removal of blood or fluid from the cul-de-sac behind the uterus. It is a gynecological test that relies on the term "culdo," which means cul-de-sac, and "centesis," which means to remove fluid from something.

- **Colposcopy.** This is a visual examination of the vagina and cervix. It relies on the root word for "vagina," which is "colpo," and the suffix "scopy," which refers to the visual examination of something.

- **Pseudocyesis.** This is a psychiatric condition in which the woman has an imagined or "false" pregnancy. It relies on the root word "cyesis," which means pregnancy, and the prefix "pseudo," which means false.

- **Embryology.** This is the study of the embryo and embryo development. It is based on the root word "embryo," which is the term for "embryo."

- **Estrogen.** This is a hormone commonly seen in the female reproductive system. It relies on the root word "estro," which means something female, and "gen," which means "substance that produces."

- **Epididymitis.** This is an inflammation of the epididymis. It is named from the root word "epdidymo" and the suffix "itis," which means inflammation.

- **Episiotomy.** This is a surgical procedure in which the perineum is cut into and repaired during the birth process. It is a bit of a misnomer as "episi" means vulva and not the perineum, while "tomy" refers to the process of cutting.

- **Fetoscope.** This is a device used to measure the heartbeat externally in the examination of a pregnant woman. It relies on the root word "feto," which means "fetus," or referring to the fetus. The suffix is "scope," which involves viewing something.

- **Galactorrhea.** This is a flowing of milk from the breasts, which may or may not be normal. It is normal during pregnancy and after giving birth, but it can also occur at other times when it is not considered normal. The term "galacto" means milk, and "rrhea" means to flow.

- **Gestational sac.** This is the small sac seen on an ultrasound in early pregnancy. It relies on the root word "gesto," which means pregnancy, or describing a pregnancy.

- **Gonad.** This is a male or female reproductive organ that produces the sperm or egg. The root word is "gon," which means "seed," so the term specifically defines the testes and the egg.

- **Gravid.** This means "pregnant" in medical terms. The word "gravid" is the root word for the entire word, although there are other terms that can be made from "gravido," including "gravidarum"(as in hyperemesis gravidarum), which is excessive vomiting in pregnancy.

- **Multigravida.** This basically means many pregnancies; it uses the prefix "multi," which means many, and "gravida," which refers to a pregnant woman.

- **Gynecology.** This is the study of diseases of the woman. It relies on the root word "gyneco," which means something related to the female or woman, and the suffix "ology," which means the study of.

- **Hymenectomy.** This is the surgical excision of the hymen. It makes use of the root word "hymen," which means hymen. The suffix means the excision of something.

- **Hysteria.** This means being anxious and irrational. It is based on the root word "hyster," which means uterus. It was once believed that anxiety and irrational thoughts were related to the female uterus.

- **Karyotype.** This is the study of the chromosomes of the fetus. It refers to the root word "karyo," which means nucleus, and the suffix "type," which means classification (or picture) of something.

- **Outer or inner labia.** This refers to the outer or inner lips of the female genitalia or vulva. The term "labi" means lip.

- **Lactating.** This refers to a woman who is breastfeeding. It relies on the root word "lacto," which means milk.

- **Leiomyoma.** This is a benign muscle tumor of the uterus. The term "leio" means smooth and "myo" means muscle. The suffix "oma" means tumor. This is a smooth muscle tumor.

- **Mammogram.** This is an X-ray picture of the breasts. The term "mammo" means breast and the suffix "gram" means record.

- **Menorrhagia.** This means excessive menstrual flow. It is based on the term "meno," which means menstruation. Another similar term is "menometrorrhagia," which relies on both the term for menstruation and the term for womb, which is "metro."

- **Endometritis.** This is an infection or inflammation of the lining of the uterus. The term "metri" refers to the uterus, while the term "endo" means in, or within.

- **Obstetrician.** This is a specialist in birth or pregnancy. The root word "obstetr" means birth or pregnancy, while "ician" refers to being a specialist in something.

- **Orchitis.** This is an inflammation or infection of the male testes. The root word "orch" or "orchi" refers to the testes, while the suffix refers to inflammation.

- **Ovum.** This is another term for "egg." It relies on the root word "ov" or "ovo" — both of which mean egg.

- **Ovarian cancer.** This refers to cancer of the ovaries. The term "ovario" means ovary, accompanied by the typical suffix "ian" or "an," which mean pertaining to.

- **Ovulation.** This is the act of releasing the egg. It relies on the prefix "ovul," which refers to the egg, while "ation" refers to the act of doing something.

- **Para.** This is the medical term referring to the number of live births. It means to bring forth or to bear.

- **Multiparous.** This refers to someone who has given birth many times. The prefix "multi" means many, while the suffix "parous" means to bring forth or to bear (as in to give birth).

- **Dyspareunia.** This means difficult or painful sexual intercourse. The medical term for intercourse is "pareunia," while "dys" means bad, painful, or difficult.

- **Antepartum.** This means before giving birth. The prefix "ante" means before, and the suffix "partum" refers directly to labor or giving birth.

- **Perineorrhaphy.** This is a surgical procedure on the perineum. The term "perineo" refers to the perineum, while the term "rrhaphy" means to suture.

- **Phallus.** This is the medical term for penis. It is based on the root word "phall," which means penis.

- **Prostatectomy.** This is the surgical removal of the prostate gland. The prefix "prostat" means prostate, and the suffix "ectomy" means to remove something.

- **Hydrosalpinx.** This is a distally blocked fallopian tube filled with serous or clear fluid. It relies on the term "hydro," which means water, and "salpinx," which refers to the fallopian tube itself.

- **Salpingitis.** This is an inflammation of the fallopian tube and relies on the root word for fallopian tube, which is "salping."

- **Spermatocele.** This is a painless, fluid-filled cyst in the long, tightly coiled tube that lies above and behind each testicle. It relies on the root word "spermat," which refers to spermatozoa or sperm cells.

- **Spermatogenesis.** This is the making of sperm cells. The term "genesis" means beginning, and "spermato" means sperm cells or spermatozoa. The root word "sperma" also refers to spermatozoa.

- **Teratogen.** This is any drug or exposure that can cause a malformation of the fetus or a birth defect. The term "terato" means malformed fetus, while the suffix "gen" means "substance that produces."

- **Testes.** These are the male gonads. The root word "test" means testes or testis.

- **Thelarche.** This is the time when a girl begins to have breasts. It is based on the root word "the," which means nipple or breast, and the suffix "arche," which means beginning.

- **Tocodynamometer.** This is a device used in labor to monitor contractions. The giveaway here is "toco," which refers to birth or labor.

- **Dystocia.** This involves a part of the infant becoming stuck in the birth canal. The prefix "dys" means, bad, painful, difficult, or abnormal, and the suffix "tocia" means birth or labor.

- **Oxytocin.** This ia drug used to stimulate labor. It relies on the prefix "oxy," which means "swift or sharp," while "tocin" means labor or birth substance.

- **Tubo-ovarian abscess.** This is an infection and abscess of the fallopian tube and ovaries. The term "tubo" refers to the tube itself, while "ovarian" refers to the ovaries.

- **Uterine fibroid.** This is a benign tumor of the uterus. It relies on the root word for uterus, which is "uter."

- **Vaginal bleeding.** This refers to bleeding coming from the vagina. The root word for vagina is "vagin," while the suffix "al" means pertaining to.

- **Vulvar cancer.** This is cancer of the external female genitalia. The term "vulv" refers to the female vulva, while "ar" is the suffix meaning pertaining to.

This was a long list of reproductive system terms, relying on the male and female reproductive system root words. As we previously mentioned, many of the root words don't make a great deal of sense because they are based upon Latin and Greek medical terms.

CHAPTER 6:

THE URINARY SYSTEM

The urinary system involves primarily the kidneys, ureters, bladder, and urethra. These will be identified in several root words based on this system. In addition, there are terms designated for specific parts of the kidneys, parts of the bladder, metabolic wastes, and urine. These, too, are included in the root words representing aspects of the urinary system.

Root Words in the Urinary System

- **Apheresis.** This is the root word for "removal."
- **Azot/o.** This is the root word for nitrogen or urea.
- **Cali/o.** This is the root word for calyx, as in the renal calyx.
- **Calic/o.** This is a root word that also means calyx.
- **Caps/o or capsul/o.** This is the root word for capsule or container.
- **Cortic/o.** This is the root word meaning "cortex" or "outer region."
- **Cyst/o.** This is used in terms related to the urinary bladder, or a sack of fluid.
- **Glomerul/o.** This is the root word for glomerulus, as is seen in the kidneys.
- **Lithotomy.** This is a suffix phrase for removal of a stone.
- **Nephr/o.** This is a root word meaning "kidney."
- **Prostat/o.** This is the root word that means the male prostate gland.
- **Ren/o.** This is the root word referring to kidney.
- **Trigon/o.** This refers to the trigone area of the bladder.

- **Uresis.** This is a suffix word that means urination.

- **Ur/o.** This refers to the urinary tract or to urine itself.

- **Ureter/o.** This refers to the ureter.

- **Urethr/o.** This refers to the urethra.

- **Uria.** This is a suffix relating to urination.

- **Uric/o.** This is a root word relating to a urine condition.

- **Urin/o.** This is a root word relating to urine.

- **Vesic/o.** This is a root word for the urinary bladder.

Putting it All Together

Here are some medical terms to remember:

- **Plasmapheresis.** This is a method of removing blood plasma from the body by withdrawing blood, separating it into plasma and cells, and transfusing the cells back into the bloodstream. It is performed to remove antibodies when treating autoimmune conditions. The term relies on the suffix "apheresis," which means "remove."

- **Azotemia.** This is a term that means urea or nitrogen in the blood and is a condition that occurs during renal failure. The root word "azot" (which means nitrogen or urea) is added to "emia," which means "blood condition."

- **Nephroblastoma.** This is a kidney cancer that consists of immature cancer cells. It relies on the root word "nephro," which means kidney, and "blastoma," which means immature tumor cells. It is a rare kidney cancer seen in children.

- **Caliceal stone.** This is a kidney stone located in the calyx of the kidney. The term "cali" refers to the renal calyx, while "eal" means relating to or pertaining to.

- **Renal capsule.** This is the outer covering of the kidneys. The term relies on the root word "ren," which means kidney and "capsul," which means capsule or container. The renal capsule is a distinct outer covering seen in all kidneys.

- **Cystoscopy.** This is a visual inspection of the urinary bladder. It relies on the root word "cysto," which means urinary bladder, and "scopy," which means a visual inspection of something.

- **Genitourinary system.** This is the system of the reproductive organs and of the urinary system. It relies on the root word "genito," which means relating to reproduction, and "urin," which relates to urine. The term "ary" means pertaining to.

- **Glomerulonephritis.** This is an infection or inflammation of the kidneys that particularly involves the glomeruli. The term "glomerulo" means glomerulus and defines the location in the kidneys where this can be seen.

- **Urethral meatus.** This is the opening to the urethra in both the male and female. The term "urethr" means "urethra" and the term "meato" refers to meatus.

- **Trigone.** This is a triangular area on the wall of the bladder. The root word is the same as the word itself; "trigon" means the trigone of the bladder.

- **Diuresis.** This is when a diuretic causes an increased flow of urine. The prefix is probably "dia," which means complete or through, while "uresis" means urination.

- **Ureteral stone.** This is a stone that has lodged in the ureter. It relies on the root word "ureter," which refers to the ureter, with "al" meaning pertaining to.

- **Polyuria.** This is excessive urination. The prefix "poly" means much or many, while "uria" refers to urination.

- **Vesicoureteral junction.** This is the connection between the bladder and the ureter. It relies on the root word "vesico," which means urinary bladder, and "ureteral," which refers to the ureters.

- **Cystocele.** This divides into "cysto/cele," and means the protrusion (herniation) of the bladder. It relies on the root word "cysto," which means bladder.

- **Cystitis.** This breaks up into "cyst/itis" and means an inflammation of the bladder. The root word "cysto" means bladder.

- **Cystolithotomy.** This divides into "cysto/lith/otomy" and means "removal of a stone in the bladder." There are two root words to know in this case: "cysto" and "lith."

- **Hydronephrosis.** This basically means "abnormal condition of water on the kidney" based on the breakdown of "hydro/nephr/osis." It is a condition where there is an obstruction of the urinary tract, leading to dilation of the calyces of the kidneys.

- **Nephritis.** This is broken down into "nephr/itis" and means "inflammation of the kidneys."

- **Nephroma.** This breaks down into "nephr/oma," which means "tumor of the kidney."

- **Cystorrhaphy.** This is divided into "cysto/rrhaphy," which means "suturing of the bladder." The root word "cysto" means bladder, while "rrhaphy" means "to suture."

- **Cystostomy.** This is divided into "cyst/ostomy," which means "creating an artificial opening into the bladder."

- **Lithotripsy.** This breaks down into "lith/otripsy" (the "surgical crushing of a stone"), which may be in the kidneys, ureter or bladder.

- **Nephrectomy.** This is divided into "nephr/ectomy" or the "excision or removal of a kidney."

- **Nephropexy.** This is divided into "nephr/opexy," which ultimately means "the surgical fixation of the kidney."

- **Nephrogram.** This breaks down into "nephr/o/gram" or a "radiographic image of the kidney."

- **Cystogram.** This divides into "cyst/o/gram," which means a "radiographic image of the bladder."

- **Dysuria.** This divides into "dys/ur/ia," or a condition of difficult or painful urination.

- **Anuria.** This involves the negation prefix of "an" and divides into "an/ur/ia," or a condition of the "absence of urine."

- **Glycosuria.** This divides into "glyc/os/ur/ia," or a condition of "sugar in the urine."

- **Hematuria.** This divides into "hemat/ur/ia," or "blood in the urine."

- **Nephrologist.** This divides into "nephr/o/log/ist," which means a specialist or "physician who specializes in disorders of the kidney."

- **Nocturia.** This is divided into "noct/ur/ia," or the condition of "night urination" — the problem of getting up and urinating in the night.

- **Oliguria.** This word breaks down into "olig/ur/ia" or "scanty urine (small amount)." The final "o" has been dropped in the prefix "oligo" so that the word makes sense.

- **Urologist.** The word divides into "ur/o/log/ist," a specialist or physician who specializes in treating diseases of the urinary tract.

- **Vesicovaginal fistula.** This has two root words "vesico" and "vagin," which breaks down as "vesico/vagin/al." This is when there is an opening between the vagina and urinary bladder.

Fortunately, there are not many words in the urinary system to memorize. If you remember the basic root words for the kidneys, bladder, ureters, and urethra, you'll have most of the words you need to recognize a urinary system word when you need to.

CHAPTER 7:

THE DIGESTIVE SYSTEM

The digestive system is a bit bigger than the urinary system, encompassing everything from the mouth to the anus. There are terms related to the digestive tract itself, as well as things like the pancreas, gallbladder, and the liver. It's a big system and there is a lot to learn.

Root Words of the Digestive System

These are the main root words (derived primarily from the Greek and Latin language) that are used in describing digestive system terminology. They may not make sense alone but, these key root words will be combined with prefixes, other root words, and suffixes, to make words that are recognizable as medical terminology.

The root words that should be memorized include the following:

- **Abdomin/o.** This is the root word referring to the abdomen.
- **An/o.** This is the root word pertaining to the anus.
- **Anthr/o.** This is any root word that pertains to the antrum of the stomach.
- **Aphth/o.** This refers to an ulcer of some kind.
- **Append/o.** This refers to the appendix.
- **Appendic/o.** This also refers to the appendix.
- **Ase.** This is a suffix that defines all enzymes, including the mouth, stomach, and pancreatic enzymes.
- **Bar/o.** This refers to either weight or pressure.

- **Bary.** This is a prefix word that also refers to weight or pressure.
- **Bil/i.** This means bile or gallbladder.
- **Bilirubin/o.** This refers to bilirubin.
- **Catharo or Cathart/o.** This refers to purging or cleansing.
- **Cec/o.** This refers to the cecum or the first part of the large bowel.
- **Cele.** This is a suffix term meaning hernia.
- **Celi/o.** This is the root word for abdomen or belly.
- **Chalasia or Chalasis.** These are suffix terms used to describe relaxation (of a viscus).
- **Chezia.** This is a suffix term related to defecation or elimination.
- **Cheil/o.** This is the root word for lip.
- **Chlorhydr/o.** This is the root word for hydrochloric acid.
- **Chol/e.** This means bile or gallbladder.
- **Cholangi/o.** This means bile or vessel.
- **Cholecyst/o.** This is the root word for gallbladder.
- **Choledoch/o.** This is the root word for common bile duct.
- **Cirrh/o.** This means orange or yellow coloration.
- **Col/o.** This refers to the colon itself.
- **Colon/o.** This also refers to the colon itself.
- **Dent/i.** This refers to the tooth or teeth.
- **Dips/o.** This refers to thirst or being thirsty.
- **Dote.** This is the suffix for "to give."
- **Duct/o.** This basically means to lead or to carry.
- **Duoden/o.** This is the root word for duodenum.
- **Emesis.** This is the suffix that means "to vomit."
- **Enter/o.** This is the root word that means intestines (generally the small intestines).
- **Epiglott/o.** This is the root word for epiglottis (in the pharynx).
- **Epithel/o.** This means epithelium but can refer to the skin itself.

- **Esophag/o.** This is the root word for esophagus.
- **Gastro.** This is the root word for stomach.
- **Gloss/o.** This is the root word for tongue.
- **Gnath/o.** This is the root word for "jaw."
- **Heli/o.** This is the root word for "ulcer."
- **Helminth.** This is the root word meaning worm.
- **Herni/o.** This is a root word that means hernia.
- **Ile/o.** This is the root word for ileum.
- **Inguin/o.** This is the root word for groin.
- **Jaund/o.** This is the root word meaning "yellow."
- **Jejun/o.** This is the root word meaning jejunum.
- **Lapar/o.** This refers to the abdominal wall or abdomen.
- **Lien/o.** This is the root word that means "spleen."
- **Nutri/o or nutrit/o.** These are the root words meaning "to nourish."
- **Omphal/o.** This is the root word for umbilicus or navel.
- **Orexia.** This is a suffix that means "appetite."
- **Pancreat/o.** This is the root word for pancreas.
- **Pepsia.** This is the suffix word for digestion.
- **Peritone/o.** This is the root word for peritoneum.
- **Phage.** This means to eat or swallow.
- **Phagia.** This is the root word for eat and swallow.
- **Pin/o.** This is the root word for "drink" or "to drink."
- **Posia.** This is the suffix term for "drinking."
- **Prandial.** This is a suffix word that means meal.
- **Proct/o.** This is the root word meaning anus or rectum.
- **Ptyl/o.** This is the root word meaning "saliva."
- **Ptysis.** This is a suffix word that means spitting.
- **Pylor/o.** This is the root word for pylorus or pyloric sphincter.

- **Sial/o.** This is the root word for saliva.

- **Sialaden/o.** This is the root word for salivary gland.

- **Sigmoid/o.** This is the root word that means sigmoid colon.

- **Splanchn/o.** This is a root word meaning viscera, or internal organs.

- **Splen/o.** This is the root word for spleen.

- **Stalsis.** This is the suffix meaning "contraction."

- **Stomia.** This is a suffix that means "condition of the mouth."

- **Stomat/o.** This is the root word for mouth.

- **Steat/o.** This is the root word for fat or sebum.

- **Viscer/o.** This is a root word for viscera, or internal organs.

- **Zym/o.** This means enzyme or ferment.

Putting it All Together

The root words themselves don't mean much until they are put together into real words related to the abdomen and digestive system. The following are words that can be made from the root words and the prefixes and/or suffixes that go with them.

Here are some words and their meaning:

- **Abdominoplasty.** This is a surgical procedure to repair tissue on the abdomen. It makes use of the root word "abdomino" and the suffix "plasty," which means surgical repair.

- **Anoscopy.** This word, by definition, means "visual examination of the anus." It involves using a device to open and visualize the tissues of the anus and is used by proctologists to evaluate anal complaints.

- **Aphthous ulcer.** This is a canker sore and literally means ulceration. It relies on the root word "aphtho," which refers to an ulcer.

- **Appendicitis.** This can use the root word "append" or "appendic," both of which mean appendix. The suffix implies an inflammation or infection of the appendix.

- **Amylase.** This is a pancreatic and oral enzyme used to digest carbohydrates. Because it ends in the suffix "ase," it is likely to be labeled an enzyme by definition.

- **Bariatric surgery.** This is the same thing as weight loss surgery and is defined as such because the root word "bary" means weight or pressure. The suffix "iatric" means "referring to or pertaining to."

- **Bilirubin.** This is a heme-based molecule made by the liver and stored in the gallbladder. It is the breakdown product of hemoglobin. The terms "bili" and bilirubin both relate to bile and the gallbladder, so this protein is named as such.

- **Cathartic.** This is a drug capable of purging or cleansing the gastrointestinal tract. It can result in vomiting or diarrhea but, based on its root term "cathart," causes purging or cleansing.

- **Ileocecal valve.** This is, by definition, a valve between the ileum and cecum in the intestinal tract. The root words "ileo" and "cec" are used to define this valve.

- **Omphalocele.** This is a condition in which a baby is born with a large herniation of abdominal contents through a defect in the umbilicus. It relies on the root words "omphalo" and "cele," which mean umbilicus and hernia, respectively.

- **Celiac disease.** This is basically a misnomer because it means "of or pertaining to the abdomen," which is fairly vague. In reality, it is a digestive problem caused by an intolerance to gluten, which results in the malabsorption of nutrients.

- **Achalasia.** This is a condition of the esophagus where the esophagus fails to relax. The term "chalasia" means (by definition) "no relaxation," which results in food building up in the esophagus during eating.

- **Hematochezia.** This literally means the defecation or elimination of blood, or bleeding in the stools. It relies on the root words "hemato," which means blood, and "chezia," which means defecation or elimination.

- **Cheilitis.** This involves inflammation of the lips and is based on the root word "cheil," which means lip and "itis," which means inflammation.

- **Achlorhydria.** This literally means "a condition of lack of hydrochloric acid" and happens when the stomach doesn't make enough acid. It breaks down into "a/chlorhydr/ia."

- **Cholelithiasis.** This basically means a condition of stones in the gallbladder. The root word "chole" means bile or gallbladder, while "litho" means stone, and "iasis" refers to having a condition.

- **Cholangiogram.** This is a dye study of the bile vessels/ducts. It relies on the root word "cholangio" with "gram," which means "to record."

- **Choledocholithiasis.** This is a stone in the common bile duct. The term "choledocho" means common bile duct, while the term "lithiasis" means the "condition of a stone."

- **Cholecystitis.** This involves an inflammation of the gallbladder. It makes use of the root word "cholecyst," which means gallbladder, and the inflammation suffix "itis."

- **Cirrhosis.** This is a term which means an abnormal condition of yellow or orange coloration, which is what is seen in cirrhosis, or liver disease.

- **Colonoscopy.** This can make use of the root word "colo" or "colono" plus the word "scope," which is a tool for visual examination.

- **Dentist.** This is a specialist who works with teeth. It makes use of the "dent" prefix, which means tooth or teeth.

- **Antidote.** This is something given to counteract a toxin. It literally means "to give against something."

- **Hepatic Duct.** This combines the root word for liver, which is "hepat," and the root word "duct," which means to lead or carry. It refers to the duct that carries bile from the liver.

- **Enterococcus.** This is a type of enteric bacterium. It relies on the root word "enter," which means intestines, and "coccus," which means berry-shaped bacterium. These are small, round bacterial organisms in the gut.

- **Epithelial cells.** These are the inner lining cells of the GI tract. The word relies on "epithel," which refers to the epithelial lining of the viscera.

- **Esophagoscopy.** This refers to a visual examination of the esophagus. The root word "esophago," means esophagus, while "scopy" refers to a visual examination of something.

- **Gastroenteritis.** This is an inflammation or infection of the gastrointestinal system, which can be divided into "gastro" for stomach, and "enter" for small intestines.

- **Glossitis.** This is the root word for tongue linked to "itis," which means inflammation. This translates into an inflammation of the tongue.

- **Micrognathia.** This is a condition of having a small jaw. The word relies on the prefix "micro," which means small, and "gnath," which refers to jaw. The term "ia" refers to the condition of.

- **Helicobacter pylori.** This is the bacterium responsible for stomach ulcers. The root word "heli" means ulcer, while the term "bacter" means "bacterium." The root word "pylor" means pylorus or pyloric sphincter, which is part of the stomach.

- **Herniorrhaphy.** This means a surgical repair of a hernia. The root word "hernio" means hernia, while the suffix "rrhaphy" means "to suture."

- **Inguinal hernia.** This is a hernia of the groin area. The term "inguin" refers to groin, while the root word "herni" refers to hernia.

- **Jaundice.** This refers to a yellowing of the skin as is seen in certain liver diseases. The term "jaundo" refers to "yellow," so this defines the clinical problem.

- **Laparotomy.** This is a surgical procedure involving entering the abdomen or abdominal wall. The term "laparo" refers to the abdominal wall or abdomen, while the suffix means "process of cutting."

- **Anorexia.** This means "no appetite," but basically refers to not being hungry. Patients with anorexia nervosa withhold food until they starve to death or become frightfully thin.

- **Pancreatitis.** This is an inflammation of the pancreas. The root word "pancreat" refers to the pancreas, while "itis" refers to inflammation.

- **Dyspepsia.** This basically means "bad digestion." The prefix "dys" means "bad, painful, difficult, or abnormal," and "pepsia" means digestion. Together it means bad digestion.

- **Peritonitis.** This is an inflammation of the peritoneum from the root word "periton" and the suffix "itis," which mean peritoneum and inflammation, respectively.

- **Macrophage.** This is a large cell in the immune system that "eats" other cells and cellular debris. It relies on the prefix "macro," which means large, and "phage," which means to eat or swallow.

- **Dysphagia.** This means difficulty eating or swallowing. The word "dys" means "bad, painful, difficult, or abnormal," while "phagia" means "a condition of eating or swallowing."

- **Pinocytosis.** This literally means "cell drinking." It refers to a process where the cell takes up small amounts of liquid using endocytosis. The term "pino" refers to "drinking," while "cytosis" refers to the condition of cells.

- **Postprandial.** This refers to the period of time after a meal. The prefix "post" means after, while the term "prandial" refers to a meal.

- **Proctologist.** This is a doctor who works on the anus or rectum. It makes use of the root word "procto," which means anus or rectum, and the suffix "logist," which means specialist.

- **Hemoptysis.** This means the spitting up of blood. The word relies on the prefix "hemo," which means blood and "ptysis," which means spitting. It can be either a GI source or respiratory source.

- **Sialadenitis.** This is, by definition, an inflammation or infection of the salivary gland. It relies on the root word "sialaden," which means salivary gland, and "itis," which refers to inflammation.

- **Flexible sigmoidoscopy.** This is a scope procedure or "visual inspection" of the sigmoid colon. It relies on the term "sigmoido," which means sigmoid colon and "scopy," which means visual inspection.

- **Splanchnic nerve.** This is a nerve that supplies innervation to the viscera or internal organs. It relies on the root word "splanchno," which means viscera or internal organs.

- **Splenomegaly.** This refers to having an enlarged spleen. The root word "spleno" is combined with "megaly," which means large or enlarged.

- **Peristalsis.** This is the contraction of the smooth muscle of the GI tract. It relies on the prefix "peri," which means surrounding, and "stalsis," which means contraction. The contraction surrounds the GI tract.

- **Xerostomia.** This means dryness of the mouth. The word "stomia" means condition of the mouth, while "xero" means dry.

- **Stomatitis.** This means an inflammation of the mouth. The word "stomat" means stomach, while the term "itis" means inflammation.

- **Steatorrhea.** This term refers to having fat in the stool. It basically means "steat," whichis fat, and "rrhea," which means flow or discharge.

- **Zymogen.** This is a precursor molecule to an enzyme. It relies on the root word "zymo," which means enzyme or ferment, and the suffix "gen," which means "substance that produces." It literally means a substance that produces an enzyme.

Now that you've "digested" all of these dizzying terms, you should feel more comfortable understanding terms related to this system. You can see where the prefixes and suffixes you've memorized in previous chapters help you to make more sense out of a great deal of root words that are related to this large system.

CHAPTER 8:

THE RESPIRATORY SYSTEM

If you feel as if you've been studying a different language, you likely have been. The bulk of the root words you have to memorize for the respiratory system (and the rest of the systems) are basically Greek or Latin, which have been modified slightly to make them root words for medical terminology. For example, "asbesto" is Greek for "a" and "sbestos." The "sbestos" word is Greek for "to quench," which together means "unquenchable." Let's dive in for a review of some more terms.

Root Words in the Respiratory System

These are the main root words used in the terms for the respiratory system:

- **Aero.** This is the root word for air.
- **Alveol/o.** This is the root word for alveolus, or air sac.
- **Arthria.** This is the root word for articulate, or "to speak distinctly."
- **Asbesto.** This is the root word for asbestos.
- **Atmo.** This means steam or vapor.
- **Auscult/o.** This is the root word for "to listen."
- **Bronch/o.** This is a root word for bronchial tube.
- **Bronchi/o.** This also means bronchial tube.
- **Bronchiol/o.** This means bronchiole or small bronchial tube.
- **Bucc/o.** This means cheek.
- **Capn/o.** This is the root word for carbon dioxide.

- **Capnia.** This is also a root word for carbon dioxide.
- **Cavo or cavito.** This means hollow cavity.
- **Constriction.** This means narrowing.
- **Ectasia or ectasis.** This means dilatation, dilation, or widening.
- **Laryngo.** This means voice box or larynx.
- **Lingu/o.** This means tongue.
- **Mediastin/o.** This is the root word for mediastinum.
- **Muc/o.** This is a root word for "mucus."
- **Mucos/o.** This is the root word for mucous membrane or mucosa.
- **Myx/o.** This is a root word that also means mucus.
- **Nas/o.** This is the root word for "nose."
- **Odont/o.** This is the root word for tooth.
- **Or/o.** This is a root word for mouth.
- **Pharyng/o.** This is the root word for throat or pharynx.
- **Phas/o.** This means speech.
- **Phasia.** This is a suffix that means speech.
- **Phon/o.** This is the root word for sound or voice.
- **Phonia.** This is a suffix word, which means sound or voice.
- **Pnea.** This is the root word for "breathing."
- **Pneum/o.** This is a root word for lung, air, or gas.
- **Pneumon/o.** This also means lung, air, or gas.
- **Pulmon/o.** This is the main root word for "lung."
- **Rhin/o.** This is the root word for nose.
- **Sinus/o.** This is the root word for "sinus."
- **Spiro.** This is the root word meaning "to breathe."
- **Stetho.** This is a root word for "chest."
- **Thorac/o.** This is another root word meaning "chest."
- **Thorax.** This is a root word that means chest or pleural cavity.

- **Tonsill/o.** This is the root word that means "tonsil."

- **Trache/o.** This is the root word for windpipe or trachea.

- **Uvul/o.** This is the root word meaning "uvula."

Putting it all Together

There are many combinations of prefixes, suffixes, and root words in the word of pulmonology, which is "the study of the lungs." The respiratory tract includes the nose, pharynx, larynx, windpipe, bronchial tree, and alveoli—all of which have root words linked to the respiratory system. When putting the above root words together with modifying words and phrases, the following complete terms can be made:

- **Aerate.** This means to give air or to draw in air. The root word is "aero" and it comes with the suffix "ate," which refers to the action of drawing in air.

- **Alveolitis.** This basically means inflammation of the alveoli of the lungs. It makes use of the root word "alveol," which means the alveolus or air sac, while "itis" means "inflammation."

- **Dysarthria.** This is a medical term that means to have difficulty speaking. It literally means a problem or difficulty with speaking distinctly. The root word "arthria" means "to speak distinctly."

- **Asbestosis.** This is a basic term in pulmonology. It comes from the obvious root word "abesto," which means "asbestos," and "osis," which means disease of, or condition. This is a lung disease that stems from exposure to asbestos.

- **Atmosphere.** This relies on the root word "atmo" and the suffix "sphere." The word means the surroundings we breathe in. The root word means "steam or vapor" and the suffix means "globe-shaped or round"—probably referring to the earth's air.

- **Auscultate.** This term relies on the root word "ausculto," which means "to listen." The suffix "ate" implies an action term.

- **Bronchoscopy.** This is a word that relies on the root word "broncho" and the suffix "scopy," which means visual examination. It is a term used to describe the action of looking down the bronchial tree with a scope.

- **Bronchiolitis.** This is an inflammation of the bronchioles or small airways. It relies on the root word "bronchiol," which means little bronchiole, and "itis," which means inflammation.

- **Buccal mucosa.** This is the mucous membrane inside the mouth. The root word is "bucc," which means mouth, and the suffix "al" means "pertaining to." The second word uses the root word "mucos," which means "mucus" or "mucous membrane."

- **Capnography.** This is a measurement of the amount of CO_2 in a person's system and is used to see if the patient is expiring CO_2. The word relies on the root word "capno," which means "carbon dioxide," and "graphy," which means the "process of recording."

- **Hypercapnia.** This literally means "high carbon dioxide" and is a condition involving an elevated CO_2 level. It is seen in respiratory failure when the person isn't breathing very much and begins to have rising CO_2 levels; it is also seen in a cardiac arrest, when the person isn't breathing.

- **Cavitary lesion.** This is a large, hollow cavity in the lung, as can be seen in certain infections and in certain lung diseases. It relies on the root word "cavito," which means hollow cavity, and "ary," which means pertaining to.

- **Thoracentesis.** This is a pulmonology term that uses two root words. It makes use of the word "thoraco," which means "chest," and the word "centesis," which means a surgical procedure to remove fluid. Together, the term means a surgical procedure to remove fluid from the thoracic cavity.

- **Bronchoconstriction.** This means a constriction or narrowing of the bronchial tree or bronchi. It relies on the term "broncho," which refers to a bronchus or the bronchial tree, and "constriction," which refers to narrowing.

- **Laryngospasm.** This involves a spasm or narrowing of the larynx or voice box. It relies on the root word "laryngo," which means voice box or larynx, as well as the word "spasm," which means the sudden contraction of muscles. Together, this refers to the spasm of the muscles of the larynx.

- **Linguist.** This is a person who studies speech and foreign languages. It relies on the root word "lingu," which means tongue, and the suffix "ist," which means "specialist."

- **Pneumomediastium.** This involves air in the mediastinal space, which is the space anterior to the heart and lungs. It can be caused by trauma to the chest that results in air leaking from the lungs into the mediastinum. It relies on the word "pneumo," which means lung, air, or gas, and the root word "mediastin," which refers to the mediastinum. The suffix "um" refers to structure, tissue, or thing.

- **Myxoid cyst.** This is a cyst that contains mucus. It relies on the root word "myx," which means mucus and the suffix "oid," which means resembling or related to. This cyst is benign and occurs on different body areas.

- **Nasopharyngitis.** This is an inflammation or infection of the nose and pharynx (or throat). It relies on two root words, "naso," which means "nose," and "pharyng," which means throat or pharynx. The suffix "itis" means inflammation.

- **Odontology.** This is the scientific study of the structure of, or diseases of, teeth. It relies on the root word "odont," which means tooth, and "ology," which means the study of.

- **Circumoral.** This means around the mouth. It relies on the prefix "circum," which means around, and "oro," which means mouth. The suffix "al" means pertaining to.

- **Aphasia.** This is a medical term which basically means "no speech." A person can have "aphasia" for any number of reasons, including lung-related and nervous system-related reasons.

- **Dysphonia.** A hoarse voice, also known as hoarseness or dysphonia, is when the voice involuntarily sounds breathy, raspy, or strained. It relies on the root word "phon," which means sound or voice, and the prefix "dys," which means bad, painful, difficult, or abnormal. The suffix "ia" means "condition." Basically, it means condition of a bad or difficult voice.

- **Apnea.** This means basically "no breathing." The root word is "pnea," which means breathing. The prefix "a" means no. A patient with apnea is not breathing at all.

- **Pneumothorax.** This is a medical condition involving having air in the pleural cavity or chest cavity. It relies on the two root words, "pneumo" and "thorax," which mean "lung, air, or gas" and "chest or pleural cavity," respectively.

- **Pneumonia.** This is an infection of the lung tissues. It is a bit of a misnomer because nothing in the word actually means this. The prefix "pneumon" means lung, air, or gas, and the suffix "ia" means condition. Together, however, they mean the lung condition involving infection of the lung.

- **Pulmonary.** This refers to anything related to the lung and is used in terms like "pulmonary abscess," "pulmonary embolism," and "pulmonary edema." The root word "pulmon" means lung, while the suffix "ary" means pertaining to. Many lung-related medical terms use this word to explain the meaning of the term and to describe it as relating to the lungs.

- **Rhinitis.** This is an inflammation or infection of the nose. It relies on the root word "rhin," which means nose and "itis," which means inflammation.

- **Rhinosinusitis.** This is a more complex term meaning an inflammation or infection of the nose and sinuses. It relies on the two root words, "rhino" and "sinus," to refer to both of these areas.

- **Inspire.** This means to breathe in. The opposite word would be to "expire," which also means "to die." The Prefixes "in" and "ex" mean "in or into" and "out or out of," respectively, and "spire" comes from the root word "spiro," which means "to breathe."

- **Spirometer.** This is a device that measures breathing. It relies on the root word "spiro" and the suffix "meter," which can refer to either a measuring device or to the act of measuringe.

- **Stethoscope.** This is a device that listens to the chest. It relies on the root word "stetho," which means chest, and the suffix "scope," which means an instrument for evaluation. This is the main device used to listen to the lungs.

- **Tonsillitis.** This is an inflammation or infection of the tonsils. It relies on the root word "tonsill," which means tonsil, and the suffix "itis," which means inflammation or infection.

- **Endotracheal intubation.** This involves placing a tube in the trachea. It relies on multiple prefixes, suffixes, and root words. The root words are "trache" (windpipe) and "tub" (tube). The prefix "endo" means within (or in), and the prefix "in" means into (or within). The suffix "eal" means pertaining to, and "ion" means the process of. This completes the breakdown of "endo/trach/eal in/tuba/tion."

- **Uvulectomy.** This is a procedure done for patients who have sleep apnea. It is done in order to improve airflow in the pharynx by removing the "uvula." The root word "uvul" means uvula, while the suffix "ectomy" means removal, excision, or resection.

As you can see, the respiratory system is big and includes things related to the oropharynx, trachea, bronchi, and lungs. This leads to a dizzying number of medical terms, which are easier to remember now that you've memorized the root words, prefixes, and suffixes related to this system.

CHAPTER 9:

THE CARDIOVASCULAR SYSTEM

The cardiovascular system involves not only the heart, but also the blood vessels (arteries and veins) and the blood system. This leads to many root words related to these body areas. There are a number of root words to memorize but, once this is done, your knowledge of the cardiovascular system should be much greater, and you will be able to combine the root words to make a wide variety of useful medical terms.

Cardiovascular System Root Words

Here are the root words that are used as part of this system:

- **Agglutin/o.** This means clumping or sticking together.
- **Aneurysm/o.** This means the widening of a blood vessel.
- **Angio.** This basically means blood vessel.
- **Aort/o.** Relating to the aorta or the largest artery in the body.
- **Aque/o.** This means water.
- **Arter/o.** This means artery.
- **Arteri/o.** This also means artery.
- **Arteriol/o.** This means arteriole or small artery.
- **Ather/o.** This means a fatty plaque or fatty substance within the blood vessels.
- **Atri/o.** This refers to the atrium, or upper chamber of the heart.
- **Cardi/o.** This refers to "heart" and is commonly used in cardiovascular terms.
- **Cholesterol/o.** This refers to "cholesterol."

- **Coagul/o.** This refers to coagulation.
- **Coron/o.** This essentially means crown or circle but refers to the coronary arteries that encircle the heart.
- **Contus/o.** This is a verb root word, which means "to bruise."
- **Cyt/o.** This refers to cell.
- **Embol/o.** This means embolus.
- **Emia.** This means blood condition and is a suffix.
- **Emic.** This means "pertaining to a blood condition."
- **Eurysm.** This means widening, as of a blood vessel.
- **Hem/o.** This means "blood."
- **Hemat/o.** This also means "blood."
- **Hemoglobin/o.** This refers to "hemoglobin."
- **Hypo.** This means under or beneath.
- **Lip/o.** This means "fat" or "lipid."
- **Myocardi/o.** This means "myocardium," or heart muscle.
- **Neutr/o.** This means neither, neutral, or neutrophil.
- **Ox/o.** This means oxygen.
- **Oxia.** This is a suffix meaning "oxygen."
- **Phleb/o.** This means "vein."
- **Puls/o or pulsat/o.** This refers to beating or "to beat."
- **Resuscit/o.** This means "to revive."
- **Rrhage.** This means a bursting forth of blood.
- **Rrhagia.** This also means a bursting forth of blood.
- **Rhythm/o.** This means rhythm.
- **Sangu/i.** This means blood.
- **Sphygm/o.** This means "pulse."
- **Sphyxia.** This means "pulse" as well.
- **Systol/o.** This refers to "contraction," as in a contraction of the heart.

93

- **Thromb/o.** This means "clot."

- **Valv/o.** This means "valve."

- **Valvul/o.** This also means "valve."

- **Varic/o.** This refers to "varicose veins."

- **Vas/o.** This refers to vessel or duct.

- **Vascul/o.** This refers to vessel (blood vessel).

- **Ven/o.** This refers to "vein."

- **Ven/i.** This also refers to "vein."

- **Venul/o.** This means "venule," or small vein.

- **Ventricul/o.** This refers to "ventricle" of either the brain or the heart.

- **Volemia.** This is a suffix meaning "blood volume."

Putting it All Together

Now that you know a number of cardiovascular root words, it is time to put them together to create words that make some sense in the world of cardiovascular medicine. Some terms will use just one root word, while others will string together several root words to make a more complicated word. Here are a few to remember:

- **Hemagglutinin.** This is something that allows for the clumping together of blood. It makes use of two main root words: "hem," which means "blood," and "agglutinin," which means clumping or sticking together.

- **Aneurysm.** This means the widening of a blood vessel. It is a simple term to remember because the root word is the same as the medical term.

- **Angiogram.** This is a test of the blood vessels, in which a dye is used to highlight the inside of the blood vessel. It relies on the root word "angio," which means "blood vessel," and "gram," which means "record." It indicates a medical test.

- **Aortic valve.** This is the valve between the heart and the aorta. It uses the root word "aort," along with the "pertaining to" suffix "ic," to make "aortic." The word "valve" comes from the root word "valv/o," which means "valve."

- **Aqueous.** This means "pertaining to water" and is easy to remember because the root word is "aqueo," which means water.

- **Arteriole.** This is also fairly simple to remember because it refers to "a small artery" and makes use of the "arter" root word and the "ole" suffix, which means small or little.

- **Atherosclerosis.** This is a medical term that refers to the presence of a fatty plaque in the blood vessels that causes a hardening of the blood vessel. The root word "athero" means a fatty substance or plaque in the blood vessel, while "sclerosis" refers to "hardening."

- **Atrioventricular node.** This is a node that connects the nerves from the atrium and the ventricle of the heart. It relies on the root word "atrio" and the root word "ventricul," with the "ar" suffix.

- **Cardiorespiratory.** This refers to the heart and lung systems together and relies on the root word "cardio," which basically means heart. The term "cardia" also refers to the heart, making this a common root word when it comes to studying or naming things related to the heart.

- **Bradycardia.** This means a slowing of the heart rate and makes use of the prefix "brady," which means "slow," and the root word "cardia," which means heart.

- **Tachycardia.** This means a quickening of the heart rate. It makes use of the prefix "tachy," which means "fast," and the root word "cardia," which means heart.

- **Cholesterol.** This is an easy word to remember as it comes from the root word "cholesterol/o" and refers directly to the substance itself.

- **Coagulation.** This means the clotting of blood in (or out of) the blood vessels. It uses the root words "coagul" and the suffix "ation," which means a process or condition.

- **Coronary.** There are a number of heart-related terms that use "coronary" in it. It comes from the root word "coron," which means circle or crown. The coronary arteries encircle the heart like a crown and give the term its meaning.

- **Contusion.** This means "a bruise" and uses the root word "contus," which means "to bruise," and the suffix "ion," which means "condition of."

- **Erythrocyte.** This means "red blood cell" and uses the prefix "erythro," which means red, and the suffix "cyte," which means cell. There are a number of words relating to different cells that use the suffix "cyte," such as "monocyte," "histiocyte," and "leukocyte."

- **Embolism.** This refers to having an "embolus" and uses the root word "embol," which means embolus.

- **Anemia.** This means low in blood and uses the two words "an," which means "no or not," and "emia," which means blood condition. Together it means "no blood."

- **Aneurysm.** This refers to a widening of a blood vessel and is related to the medical term "aneurysmo" and the medical term "eurysm," both of which mean a widening of a blood vessel.

- **Hemolysis.** This means a breakdown of blood. It relies on the medial term "hemo," which means blood, and the suffix "lysis," which refers to a separation or breakdown of something.

- **Hematology.** This is the study of blood. It is based on the root word "hemato," which means "blood," and "logy," which means the study of something. Many blood conditions and blood terms use this root word.

- **Hemoglobinopathy.** This is a disease of abnormal hemoglobin. It relies on the root word "hemoglobino," which means hemoglobin, and "pathy," which means disease or emotion.

- **Hypoxia.** This uses the prefix "hypo," which means under or beneath, and the root word "oxia," which means "oxygen." Together, it means low oxygen levels. The term "hypo" can be used in several medical terms, such as "hypovolemia," which means low blood volume, and "hypotension," which means low blood pressure.

- **Lipodystrophy.** This is an abnormality of the lipids. It relies on the medical root word "lipo," along with "dys" and "trophy." The term "lipo" means lipid, the term "dys" means bad or abnormal, and the term "trophy" means condition of.

- **Myocarditis.** This means an inflammation of the heart muscle and uses the root word "myocardio," which refers to the heart muscle, and the suffix "itis," which means inflammation of.

- **Oximetry.** This is a measurement of the oxygen levels in the blood and is made from the words "ox" for "oxygen," and "metry" for the process of measuring. Together, it means a test that measures oxygen levels.

- **Phlebotomy.** This refers to entering a vein to get blood. The root word "phlebo" means "vein," while the suffix "tomy" means the "process of cutting." Technically, phlebotomy does not necessarily involve a cutting of the veing—just entering it. The term does, however, make some sense.

- **Pulsatile.** This refers to a mass that has a pulse, such as an aneurysm. It makes use of the root word "pulsat," which means beating or "to beat," and the suffix "ile."

- **Resuscitation or Cardiopulmonary resuscitation (CPR).** This makes use of the root word "resuscit," which means "to revive," and "ation," which refers to the process of. "Cardiopulmonary" refers to both the heart and the lungs.

- **Hemorrhage.** This means the bursting forth of blood. It uses the two root words "hemo" and "rrhage," which is a bit redundant, but makes clear that the person is having a flow of blood bursting forth from somewhere.

- **Dysrhythmia.** This means an abnormal or bad rhythm and makes use of the root word "rhythm" and the prefix "dys," which means bad. The suffix "ia," refers to the state or condition of something.

- **Exsanguinate.** This refers to the losing of a large amount of blood, or "bleeding out of all of the blood." It uses the terms "ex," which means "out or away from," "sangui," which refers to blood, and the suffix "ate," which refers to the process of.

- **Sphygmomanometer.** This is another term for a device that measures blood pressure. It uses the medical root word "sphygmo," which means pulse, and "manometer," which refers to the measuring device itself.

- **Asphyxia.** This is a bit of a misnomer because it refers to a complete lack of oxygen, but the medical term literally means "no pulse." The term doesn't exactly translate to its meaning.

- **Systolic blood pressure.** The term "systol" means contraction, so it refers to the number or pressure of the blood vessels when the heart is contracting (as opposed to the diastolic blood pressure, which refers to the blood pressure when the heart isn't contracting). The term "diastolic" means referring to the pressure of the heart when the contraction is complete, as the prefix "dia" means through or complete.

- **Thrombosis.** This refers to a blood clot. The root word "thromb" refers to clot, and "osis" refers to a disease or abnormal condition of something.

- **Valvulotomy.** This refers to a surgery done by making one or more incisions at the edges of the commissure formed between two or three valves so as to relieve constriction (such as occurs in valvular stenosis). It makes use of the word "valvulo," which means valve. The term "tomy" refers to the surgery itself.

- **Varicosity.** This refers to a varicose vein and makes use of the term "varico," which means varicose vein, and has the suffix "ity," which refers to the condition.

- **Vasoactive.** This refers to a drug that affects the pressure of the arteries or veins. It makes use of the root word "vaso," which means vessel or duct, and the word "active," which implies its activity against the blood vessel.

- **Vasculitis.** This is an inflammation of a blood vessel. The root word in this case is "vascul," with the typical inflammatory suffix "itis."

- **Venule.** This can refer to any of the root words "veni," "veno," or "venul," all of which refer to veins. The direct meaning of the word is "small vein."

While there are a lot of possible medical terms that come from these root words, there are just a few to actually memorize. Many of the root words in the cardiovascular system (like cholesterol) are easily recognized.

CHAPTER 10:

THE LYMPHATIC SYSTEM & IMMUNITY

Lymphatic System and Immune System Root words

In addition to introducing some prefixes and suffixes in this chapter, we will also list the main root words that help define most of the terminology used in these areas. Here are some common root words you might encounter:

- **Aden/o.** This is a root word meaning gland.
- **Adenoid/o.** This is an obvious root word for "adenoids."
- **Diaphor/o.** This is a root word that means "to sweat."
- **Hidr/o.** This is a root word meaning "sweat."
- **Home/o.** This is a root word or prefix meaning constant, sameness, or unchanging.
- **Immun/o.** This is the root word for immune, safety, or protection.
- **Lymph/o.** This is a root word for lymph.
- **Lymphaden/o.** This is a root word meaning lymph node or lymph gland.
- **Lymphangi/o.** This is a root word meaning "lymph vessel."
- **Poiesis.** This is a suffix that means "formation."
- **Poietin.** This is a root word that means "substance that forms."
- **Seb/o.** This is a root word for "sebum."
- **Sebace/o.** This is a root word that also means sebum.
- **Thym/o.** This is a root word that means "thymus gland."
- **Vaccin/o.** This is a root word meaning vaccine.

- **Zyme.** This is a suffix that means "enzyme."

Putting it All Together

Some of the above terms make some sense, as they are similar to the glands they represent. Other terms are more confusing, as they are based on the Latin or Greek word for something that doesn't appear to be related. The following are terms that use prefixes, root words, and suffixes to make real medical terms used in the discussion of the immune system and the lymphatic system:

- **Adenocarcinoma.** This is a cancerous tumor that arises in glandular cells. The root word "adeno" means gland, and "carcinoma" refers to something being cancerous.

- **Adenoiditis.** This is an inflammation of the adenoid gland in the nasopharynx. The root word "adenoid" means "adenoid glands," while the suffix means, of course, inflammation.

- **Diaphoresis.** This means to sweat all over. The root word "diaphor" means to sweat. Unlike the term "hyperhidrosis" (to be discussed below), this term means to sweat all over—rather than just from the sweat glands of the armpits and groin (as is seen in "hyperhidrosis").

- **Hyperhidrosis.** This is a medical term for excessive sweating. The prefix "hyper" means above or over, and "hidr" means to sweat. The ending "osis" refers to a pathological condition. This basically refers to excess sweating by the armpit and groin sweat glands.

- **Homeopathy.** This is a branch of study that gives treatments that are the "same" as the thing a person cannot tolerate. The intention is, by giving small doses of such a substance to that person, to build up their tolerance levels. The root word is "homeo" and the suffix is "pathy," which means disease state.

- **Immunology.** This is the study of the immune system. Quite simply, the term "immun" means immune, safety, or protection, while "logy" means the study of. This basically comes together to mean the study of the immune system.

- **Lymphocyte.** This is a white blood cell found in the lymph bodes and blood stream. The root word is "lympho," which means lymph, and "cyte" is the suffix, which means cell.

- **Lymphadenitis.** This is an inflammation or infection of a lymph node. It is based on the root word "lymphaden," which means lymph node, and "itis," which means inflammation.

- **Lymphangitis.** This is an infection of the lymph vessels and results in the typical "red streaks" seen in certain infections. It relies on the terms "lymphangi" and the inflammation suffix ("itis") to make the complete word.

- **Erythropoiesis.** This is the act of making new red blood cells in the bone marrow. The root words are "erythro" for "red" (as in a red blood cell), and "poiesis," which means "formation."

- **Erythropoietin.** This is a substance that helps to form red blood cells by being secreted during times when a low red blood cell count is noted. The root words are "erythro" for "red" and "poietin," which means "substance that forms."

- **Sebaceous glands.** These are glands that make sebaceous material in the skin. The root word/prefix is "seb," which means "sebum."

- **Thymus.** This is based on the root word "thym," which is the gland in the chest that helps to mature T cells in the immune system.

- **Vaccination.** This is the word used to describe giving a shot to boost the immune response toward an antigen. The root word is "vacc," which means vaccine.

- **Proenzyme.** This is a precursor molecule to an enzyme. Pepsinogen, for example, is the proenzyme for pepsin. The root word is "pro," which means "before," and "zyme" is a suffix meaning enzyme.

While there were two systems to memorize in this chapter, the number of root words/terms was small, and the words that can be made from them is fairly simple to put together.

CHAPTER 11:

THE ENDOCRINE SYSTEM

The endocrine system involves all of the hormones, as well as the glands that make hormones. This includes the pituitary gland, the adrenal gland, the endocrine pancreas, thyroid gland, the parathyroid glands, and others. Most of the root words you'll learn are recognizable as glands you probably already know about.

Endocrine System Root words

In this section, we will list the main root words that help define most of the terminology used in the endocrine system. Here are some common root words you might encounter:

- **Adren/o.** This is the root word for adrenal gland.
- **Adrenal/o.** This is a root word that means "adrenal gland."
- **Crin/o.** This is the root word meaning "to secrete."
- **Crine.** This is a suffix term meaning to secrete or separate.
- **Gluc/o.** This is a root word that means sugar or glucose.
- **Glyc/o.** This is a root word for sugar or glucose.
- **Glycogen/o.** This is a root word for glycogen or animal starch.
- **Glycos/o.** This is a root word meaning sugar or glucose.
- **Hormon/o.** This is a root word for "hormone."
- **Insulin/o.** This is a root word for insulin.
- **Pineal/o.** This is a root word that means the pineal gland.
- **Pituitar/o.** This is a root word that means the pituitary gland.

- **Thyr/o.** This is a root word that means thyroid gland or shield (referring to the shape of the gland).
- **Thyroid/o.** This is a root word meaning "thyroid gland."

Putting it All Together

The following are terms that use prefixes, root words, and suffixes to make real medical terms used in the discussion of the endocrine system:

- **Adrenalectomy.** This is a removal of the adrenal gland. There are two root words for "adrenal gland." The first is "adreno" and the second is "adrenalo." Both mean adrenal gland. The term "ectomy" refers to the removal of something.

- **Endocrinology.** This makes use of the prefix "endo," meaning "in," "crin," which means "to secrete," and "ology," which is the study of something. Together, this means the study of secreting in something, or the study of hormones and the endocrine system.

- **Exocrine.** This refers to a gland that secretes a substance that is released through the epithelial cells and not directly to the bloodstream. It relies on the term "exo," which means outside of, and "crine," which means to secrete or separate.

- **Glucometer.** This is a device that measures the blood sugar content in the bloodstream. The term "gluco" means sugar or glucose, and "meter" means to measure.

- **Glycolysis.** This involves the breakdown of glucose in metabolism. The term "glyco" refers to glucose or sugar, while "lysis" means the breakdown of something.

- **Glycogen.** This is fairly easy to remember because the root word and the meaning of the word are the same. Glycogen is basically animal starch stored in the liver.

- **Glycosuria.** This mean spilling or secreting glucose in the urine. It comes from the root word "glycos," which means sugar or glucose, and "uria," which means "related to urination."

- **Hormone.** This is the word for the substance secreted by a gland into the bloodstream, usually in order to act on a distant site. The root word is simply "hormon."

- **Insulinoma.** This is a benign insulin-secreting tumor. It is derived from the root word "insulin," which means insulin, and "oma," which refers to it being a tumor.

- **Pineal gland.** This is a small gland located in the brain that secretes melatonin for the circadian rhythm and for sleep. The root word is "pineal," which makes it easy to remember.

- **Pituitary gland.** This is the gland in the base of the brain that secretes a number of endocrine hormones. The root word is "pituitar" with the simple suffix of "y."

- **Thyroid gland.** This is the butterfly-shaped gland in the anterior surface of the neck that produces the thyroid hormone. The root word is "thyr" with the suffix "oid," meaning pertaining to. The root word "thyr" also means "shield," which is the approximate appearance of the gland on the anterior portion of the chest.

- **Thyroidectomy.** This is the removal of the thyroid gland. The term "thyroid" means "thyroid gland," while the suffix "ectomy" refers to the removal of something.

- **Thyroiditis.** This is a type of autoimmune disease that affects the thyroid gland. It may cause enlargement (a goiter), and although it occasionally may cause temporary overactivity of the thyroid gland (hyperthyroidism), it usually causes permanent underactivity (hypothyroidism).

- **Hyperparathyroidism.** This is divided into "hyper/para/thyroid/ism." It refers to overactivity and the growth of the parathyroid gland or glands.

- **Hyperthyroidism.** This is the overproduction of thyroid hormones.

- **Hypothyroidism.** This is underproduction, or ineffectiveness, of thyroid hormones.

- **Parathyroidectomy.** This is an operation to remove a parathyroid gland.

Now that you are highly familiar with prefixes and suffixes, you should be able to use the root words you've learned in order to make the medical terminology related to the endocrine system.

CHAPTER 12:

THE MUSCULOSKELETAL SYSTEM

The musculoskeletal system (the muscular and skeletal system) is studied as one system here because the terms often go together. Muscles are often named for the bones they attach to and so there is a lot of overlap between the skeletal system and the muscular system. As you'll discover, other muscles are named for their shape or size, the same being true for some bones. An example is "clavicle," which is a diminutive for "clavus," which is a Latin wordfor "nail." There are a lot of words to remember in this chapter, but they will give you an excellent understanding of the muscles and bones in the body.

Musculoskeletal Root Words

Here are some common musculoskeletal root words and what they mean. Later in this chapter, we will use them with the appropriate prefixes and suffixes (if applicable) in order to better understand where the different terms come from:

- **Acetabul/o.** This basically means acetabulum, which is the medical term for the hip socket.

- **Acromi/o.** This is the root word for acromion, which is an extension of the shoulder bone.

- **Acro.** This refers to the extremities but can also mean the extreme point or top.

- **Aponeuro.** This refers to the aponeurosis, or a type of tendon in the body.

- **Arthr/o.** This refers to a joint. There are many musculoskeletal terms that use this root word.

- **Articulo.** This also refers to a joint in the body.

- **Axillo.** This is an anatomic term referring to the axilla, or underarm area.
- **Axi/o.** This is an anatomic term referring to the axial, as in the axial skeleton.
- **Bunion/o.** This means bunion, a bump on the proximal MP joint of the great toe.
- **Burs/o.** This means "bursa," or a fluid-filled sac near a joint or tendon.
- **Calcaneo.** This refers to the calcaneus, or heel bone.
- **Carp/o.** This refers to the wrist joint or "carpal" bones.
- **Caud/o.** This refers to the tail or the lower part of the body.
- **Chir/o.** This is a root word meaning "hand."
- **Chondr/o.** This is a root word meaning cartilage.
- **Cephal/o.** This is a root work meaning "head" or "toward the head."
- **Cineo.** This is a root word meaning "movement."
- **Clavicul/o.** This means clavicle or collar bone.
- **Cleid/o.** This also means clavicle or collar bone.
- **Coccyg/o.** This refers to the tail bone or coccyx.
- **Corpor/o.** This means "body" or "corpus."
- **Cost/o.** This is a root word that means "rib."
- **Cox/o.** This is a root word that means "hip."
- **Crani/o.** This is a root word that means "skull."
- **Cubit/o.** This refers to the elbow or forearm and is a root word.
- **Dactyl/o.** This is a root word meaning fingers or toes.
- **Dors/o.** This refers to the back, such as the back of the body.
- **Fasci/o.** This is a root word meaning "fascia," or a membrane separating tissues of the body.
- **Femor/o.** This is a root word meaning "thigh bone," or "femur."
- **Fibr/o.** This is a root word meaning fiber.
- **Fibros/o.** This is a root word meaning fibrous connective tissue.
- **Fibul/o.** This is a root word meaning fibula.
- **Flex/o.** This means "to bend."

- **Histo.** This is a root word meaning "tissue."
- **Histio.** This is a root word meaning "tissue."
- **Humer/o.** This means upper arm bone, or "humerus."
- **Ili/o.** This refers to the ilium.
- **Ischi/o.** This refers to the ischium, which is a part of the pelvic bones.
- **Kyph/o.** This is a root word meaning "humpback."
- **Lamin/o.** This is a root word meaning "lamina."
- **Leiomy/o.** This is a root word meaning "smooth muscle."
- **Ligament/o.** This basically means "ligament."
- **Listhesis.** This is a suffix that means "slippage," as of the vertebral bodies.
- **Lord/o.** This means "swayback."
- **Lumb/o.** This means lower back or loin.
- **Malleol/o.** This refers to the malleolus of the ankle.
- **Mandibul/o.** This refers to the lower jaw bone.
- **Mastoid/o.** This refers to the mastoid process behind the ear.
- **Maxill/o.** This refers to the upper jaw bone.
- **Mel/o.** This refers to a limb or limbs.
- **Ment/o.** This can refer to the mind or to the chin.
- **Metacarp/o.** This refers to the hand bones.
- **Metatars/o.** This refers to the foot bones.
- **Motor.** This is a suffix referring to "movement."
- **Muscul/o.** This refers to a muscle or muscles.
- **My/o.** This refers to muscle or muscles.
- **Myom/o.** This refers to a muscle tumor.
- **Myos/o.** This refers to a muscle or muscles.
- **Olecran/o.** This refers to the tip of the elbow, or "olecranon process."
- **Om/o.** This refers to the "shoulder."
- **Ossicul/o.** This refers to a small bone or "ossicles."

- **Oste/o.** This refers to bone.

- **Ostosis.** This is a suffix that means "condition of bone."

- **Patell/a.** This refers to the kneecap.

- **Patell/o.** This refers to the kneecap.

- **Pect/oro.** This refers to "chest."

- **Pelv/i.** This refers to the pelvis or hip bone.

- **Pelv/o.** This refers to the pelvis or hip bone.

- **Ped/o.** This can refer to either a child or a "foot."

- **Perone/o.** This refers to the fibula.

- **Phren/o.** This can mean diaphragm or mind.

- **Plant/o.** This refers to the bottom of the foot.

- **Pod/o.** This refers to the foot or feet.

- **Poster/o.** This refers to the posterior part, or behind.

- **Pub/o.** This refers to the pubis or anterior part of the pelvic bone.

- **Rachi/o.** This refers to the spinal column or vertebrae.

- **Radi/o.** This can refer to the lateral lower arm bone or to X-rays.

- **Rhabdomy/o.** This refers to striated or skeletal muscle.

- **Sacr/o.** This refers to the sacrum, which is part of the pelvic structures.

- **Sarc/o.** This refers to connective tissue.

- **Scapul/o.** This refers to the scapula.

- **Skelet/o.** This refers to the skeleton.

- **Spondyl/o.** This is a root word meaning vertebra.

- **Sterno.** This refers to the sternum or breastbone.

- **Syndesm/o.** This refers to ligament.

- **Synov/o.** This refers to the synovium, or the sheath around a tendon.

- **Tal/o.** This is the root word for talus.

- **Tars/o.** This is the root word for tarsus, ankle, or hindfoot.

- **Ten/o.** This is a root word for tendon.

- **Tendon/o.** This is a root word for tendon.

- **Tibi/o.** This is the root word for tibia.

- **Uln/o.** This is the root word for ulna.

- **Ventr/o.** This means the ventral or anterior side of the body.

- **Vertebr/o.** This is the root word for vertebra or vertebral.

Putting it all Together

All of these root words are related to the musculoskeletal system (although a few are related to direction and location, which are commonly used in the musculoskeletal system). It's time to put it all together to make actual medical terms based on these root words, prefixes, and suffixes:

- **Acetabulum.** This is the hip socket joint, and it comes from the root word "acetabulo" and the suffix "um," which means structure, tissue, or thing.

- **Acromion.** This is an extension of the shoulder bone and comes from the root word "acromio" and the suffix "n," which means structure, tissue, or thing.

- **Aponeurosis.** This is a type of tendon in the body and comes from the root word "aponeuro" and the suffix "sis," which means state or condition.

- **Arthralgia**. This means joint pain. It comes from the words "arthro" and "algia." Algia means pain, so the combination "arthr/algia" means joint pain.

- **Articular**. This refers to a joint surface and basically means "of or pertaining to a joint." The root word is "articulo" and the suffix is "ar," which means "pertaining to."

- **Axillary**. This is anything that refers to the axilla or underarm. The root word "axillo" is combined with "ary," which means "of or pertaining to."

- **Bunionectomy**. This is a surgical procedure that removes bunions. The root word "buniono" is combined with "ectomy," which means removal or excision.

- **Bursitis**. This is an inflammation of the bursa, which is a fluid-filled sac near a joint or tendon. The root word "burso" is combined with the suffix "itis," which means inflammation.

- **Calcaneofibular ligament**. This combines two root words "calcaneo" and "fibulo." It uses the "ar" ending (pertaining to) and means pertaining to the calcaneus and fibula, or a ligament that connects the two bones.

- **Carpometacarpal joint**. This refers to the wrist joint and uses two root words: "carpo" and "metacarpo," along with the "al" suffix. It refers to the carpal or wrist bones and the metacarpal bones in the hand.

- **Caudal**. This refers to something closer the tail or the lower part of the body. It takes the "caudo" root word and adds the "al" suffix to it.

- **Chiropractor**. This is a person who uses "hands-on" therapy to correct musculoskeletal problems. The root word "chiro" is linked to this word, which means "hand."

- **Costochondritis**. This is an inflammation of the costochondral joints and means the joints in the chest related to the ribs. The root words "chondro" and "costo" are in it, which mean cartilage and rib, respectively.

- **Cephalopelvic disproportion**. This is actually an obstetric term that is based on the musculoskeletal system. It uses two root words "cephalo" and "pelvi," along with the suffix "ic," which means pertaining to. It pertains to the fetal head not fitting in the female pelvic inlet at the time of birth.

- **Sternocleidomastoid muscle**. This is a muscle that connects the collar bone to the mastoid process. It makes use of four root words: "sterno," "cleido," and "mastoid" in the first word, and "muscl" in the second word.

- **Coccygeal**. This is a word that uses "coccyg" and "eal," which means of or pertaining to the tailbone or coccyx.

- **Coxofemoral joint**. This is another name for the hip joint. It uses the root words "coxo" and "femor," which mean hip and thigh bone, respectively. Together, they define a joint that connects these two structures.

- **Craniofacial surgery**. This surgery is done on either the face or the skull. It makes use of the root words "cranio" and "facial." The term "cranio" is the root word meaning skull.

- **Antecubital fossa**. This is the space in front of the elbow joint. "Ante" means before and "cubital" means pertaining to the elbow or forearm.

- **Polydactyly.** This means having more than the correct number of fingers or toes. It makes use of the prefix "poly" and the root word "dactyl." The suffix "y" is added to mean a "process or condition." The prefix means "much or many."

- **Dermatomyositis.** This is a condition involving inflammation of the skin and muscles. It makes use of the root words "dermato" and "myos," as well as the "itis" suffix.

- **Fascial plane.** This is a plane or space between connective tissues. It makes use of the root word "fasci," which refers to the membranes separating tissues of the skin.

- **Fibromyalgia.** This is a condition of the muscles and "fibrous" tissue of the skin, which involves pain. It makes use of the root words "fibro" and "myo," with the suffix "algia." Fibro means fiber, indicating that it is not just the muscles that are painful in this disorder.

- **Histiocyte and Histology.** These make use of the root words "histio" and "histo," which both mean tissues. Histology is a study of the tissues of the body under the microscope (it makes use of the suffix "ology" or "logy," which means the study of). Histiocyte is a type of tissue-based immune cell. It makes use of the suffix "cyte," which means cell.

- **Humerus.** This is the bone in the upper arm that is based on the root word "humer" and the suffix "us."

- **Iliofemoral bypass.** This is surgery to bypass blockages in the upper legs. It uses the root words "ilio" and "femoro," which mean the ilium and the femur, respectively, and uses the suffix "us."

- **Ischial tuberosity.** This is a protuberance of the ischium, which is part of the pelvic bone structures.

- **Kyphosis.** This is the medical term for having a humpback and relies on the root word "kypho" and the suffix "osis," which means an abnormal condition.

- **Leiomyoma.** This is a benign smooth muscle tumor, usually affecting the uterus. It makes use of the root word "leiomy" and the suffix "oma," which means tumor. It basically means smooth muscle tumor.

- **Spondylolisthesis.** This means a forward slip of one vertebra of the spinal column relative to another. It makes use of the term "spondyl," which means vertebra, and "listhesis," which means slippage.

- **Lordosis**. This is the medical term meaning having a "swayback," or an abnormal curvature of the back in which the back is convex in shape. It is the opposite of "kyphosis."

- **Lumbosacral**. This is a term referring the lower back and sacrum. It makes use of the root words "lumbo" and "sacr," with the suffix "al" meaning pertaining to.

- **Mandibulofacial dysostosis**. This is also referred to as Treacher-Collins syndrome, which makes use of the root word "mandibulo" and "facial." Dysostosis is an abnormal condition of the bones and makes use of the root word "oste."

- **Maxillofacial surgeon**. This is a doctor who works on the face. "Maxillo" is the root word for upper jaw bone.

- **Metatarsalgia**. This is a pain in the metatarsal region of the foot. It makes use of the term "metatars," which refers to the foot bones and "algia," which means pain.

- **Olecranon bursitis**. This is a medical term referring to an inflammation or infection of the olecranon bursa. A bursa is a fluid-filled sac, while the term "olecran" refers to the tip of the elbow.

- **Osteomyelitis**. This is an infection of the bone. It makes use of the root word "osteo," which means bone, and "myel," which means bone marrow. The suffix "itis" refers to an inflammation or infection.

- **Dysostosis**. This means an abnormal formation of bone. "Dys" is a prefix meaning bad, painful, difficult, or abnormal and "ostosis" means condition of bone.

- **Patellofemoral syndrome**. This is an abnormality of the kneecap and makes use of the root words "patello" and "femor," which mean kneecap and femur, respectively.

- **Pectoral muscles**. These are chest muscles and are identified by the root word "pector," which means chest.

- **Pedometer**. This is a device that measures a person's steps. It relies on the root word "pedo," which means foot, and "meter," which means a "device that measures something."

- **Peroneal nerve**. This is a nerve near the fibula and is described as such because of its location. The root word "perone" means near the fibula.

- **Plantar fasciitis**. This is an inflammation of the plantar fascia, which is located on the sole of the foot. The term relies on the root word "plant," which means the bottom of the foot. Fasciitis uses "fasci" and "itis" to describe an inflamed membranous connective tissue.

- **Podiatrist**. This is a person who treats feet disorders. The root word "pod" refers to feet and "iatrist" refers to the specialist or doctor who does this work.

- **Pubococcygeus muscle**. This is the hammock-shaped muscle, found in both sexes, that stretches from the pubic bone to the coccyx (tail bone), forming the floor of the pelvic cavity. It relies on the root words "pubo" and "coccyg" to refer to the pubic bone and the coccyx.

- **Rhabdomyolysis**. This refers to a breakdown of striated muscle and muscle proteins in the bloodstream. It comes from the root word "rhabdomyo" and the suffix "lysis," which means a breakdown, separation, destruction, or loosening.

- **Sarcoma**. This is a connective tissue cancer. It relies on the root word "sarc," which means connective tissue, and the suffix "oma," which means tumor.

- **Skeletal dysplasia**. This refers to an abnormal growth of the skeleton. It relies on the root word "skelet," which refers to the skeleton.

- **Synovial sheath**. This is the covering around a tendon. It relies on the root word "synov," which means synovium, or "sheath around a tendon."

- **Anterior talofibular ligament**. This is an "anterior" ligament that connects the talus and the fibula by making use of the root words "talo" and "fibul," along with the suffix "ar."

- **Tenosynovitis**. This is an inflammation of the sheath around a tendon and makes use of both the root word "teno" and the root word "synov" to make the medical term.

- **Intervertebral space**. This is the space between the vertebrae and refers to the prefix "inter," which means between, and the root word "vertebr," which means vertebra. The suffix "al" completes the term.

This represented a lot of terms to memorize but, if you know things like directional prefixes and the typical suffixes, you can easily get at least some idea of what a musculoskeletal medical term means.

CHAPTER 13:

THE SPECIAL SENSES

The special senses refer to the eyes and ears primarily (or the special senses of vision and hearing). Many of these terms will be familiar to you as they represent common terms (like acoustics, which is a term related to hearing). Vision-related terms are a little more difficult as there are terms for the parts of the eye that aren't used in everyday English. Memorize the root words and be prepared to put them all together at the end of the chapter.

Root Words in the Special Senses

These are some ear and eye terms that need to be memorized. Many come from the Greek and Latin language, as words related to these terms come from a time when these languages were the basis of medical terms:

- **Acous/o.** This is a root word for hearing.
- **Acoust/o.** This is a root word for sound or hearing.
- **Acusis.** This is a root word for hearing and is often used as a suffix.
- **Ambly/o.** This is a root word for dim or dull.
- **Anis/o.** This is the root word meaning unequal.
- **Audi/o.** This is a root word for hearing.
- **Audit/o.** This is another root word for hearing.
- **Aur/o.** This is a root word meaning ear.
- **Auricul/o.** This is a root word meaning ear.

- **Blephar/o.** This is a root word meaning "eyelid."
- **Cerumin/o.** This is the root word for cerumen or earwax.
- **Choroid/o.** This is the root word for the choroid layer of the eye.
- **Cochle/o.** This is the root word for cochlea, or the inner part of the ear.
- **Conjunctiv/o.** This is the root word for conjunctiva, or the whites of the eyes.
- **Cor/o.** This is a root word for pupil.
- **Core/o.** This is a root word for pupil.
- **Corne/o.** This is a root word that means cornea.
- **Cusis.** This is a suffix meaning hearing.
- **Cycl/o.** This is a root word meaning ciliary body of the eye.
- **Dacry/o.** This is the root word meaning tear.
- **Dacryoaden/o.** This is the root word that means tear gland.
- **Dacryocyst/o.** This is the root word meaning tear sac or lacrimal sac.
- **Echo.** This is the root word meaning "reflected sound."
- **Fovea/o.** This is a root word meaning small pit or depression.
- **Goni/o.** This is a root word meaning "angle."
- **Ir/o.** This is a root word that means iris, or the colored part of the eye.
- **Irid/o.** This is a root word for the iris, or the colored part of the eye.
- **Is/o.** This means same or equal.
- **Kerat/o.** This is the root word meaning cornea. It can also mean hard or horny tissue.
- **Lacrim/o.** This is the root word for tear duct, tear, or lacrimal duct.
- **Mydr/o.** This is the root word meaning "wide."
- **Myring/o.** This is the root word for tympanic membrane, or eardrum.
- **Ocul/o.** This is a root word for "eye."
- **Ophthalm/o.** This is a root word for "eye."
- **Opia.** This is a suffix term that refers to an eye condition.
- **Opsia.** This is a suffix term that refers to a vision condition.

- **Opt/o.** This is a root word for eye or vision.

- **Optic/o.** This is a root word for eye or vision.

- **Ot/o.** This is a root word that pertains to the ear.

- **Otia.** This is a suffix that means ear condition.

- **Palpebr/o.** This is a root word meaning eyelid.

- **Phaco.** This is a root word meaning the lens of the eye. It can also be spelled "phako."

- **Phot/o.** This is the root word for "light."

- **Pupill/o.** This is the root word meaning "pupil."

- **Retin/o.** This is the root word meaning "retina."

- **Scler/o.** This is the root word for the sclera, which is the white of the eye.

- **Staped/o.** This is the root word meaning the "stapes," or middle ear bone.

- **Tympan/o.** This is the root word for the tympanic membrane, or eardrum.

- **Uve/o.** This is the root word for "uvea," or the vascular layer of the eye.

- **Vitre/o.** This is a root word for the "vitreous body of the eye."

Putting it All Together

It is not enough to learn the terms in the absence of the prefixes and suffixes that give them some meaning. In the real world, medical terms are based on root words. However, they are only sometimes based solely on the root word; usually there is some kind of modification. For this reason, we will discuss some terms that are used in modern-day medical terminology in the field of ophthalmology and diseases of the ear. Here are some helpful terms:

- **Acoustic.** This is a term that means "pertaining to hearing." It relies on the root word "acous," which means hearing, and the "ic" suffix. Another root word that may apply is "acoust."

- **Hyperacusis.** This is a debilitating disease in which the patient experiences an increased sensitivity to sounds of certain frequencies. It relies on the root word "hyper," which means "high or above," and the suffix "acusis," which means hearing.

- **Amblyopia.** This is a condition of poor vision in one eye because of a disconnect between the eye and the brain. It relies on the root word "ambly," which means dim or dull, and "opia," which means a condition of the eye.

- **Anisocoria.** This is a condition of unequal pupils. It relies on the prefix "aniso," which means unequal, and "coria," which means relating to the pupil.

- **External auditory canal.** This is the outer ear canal. It relies on the term "audit," which means hearing, and "ary," which means pertaining to. The prefix "audi" could also be in this word.

- **Auricle.** This is the external part of the ear that is visible. It relies on the term "aur," which means "ear," and "icle," which means "small."

- **Auricular cartilage.** This is the cartilage that makes up the auricle or external ear. It relies on the root word "auricul," which means ear, and the "ar" suffix.

- **Blepharospasm.** This is a spasm of the eyelid. The term "blepharo" means "eyelid," while "spasm" means a sudden contraction of muscles.

- **Ceruminectomy.** This is a word describing the removal or "excision" of the cerumen of the ear, which is the earwax. The term "cerumin" means earwax.

- **Cochlear implant.** This is an artificial implant placed in the cochlea, or inner ear, for the treatment of deafness. The root word "cochle" means inner ear or cochlea.

- **Conjunctivitis.** This is a common inflammation of the whites of the eyes and the clear covering over it. The term "conjunctiv" means the conjunctiva of the eye.

- **Corneal abrasion.** This is a scratch on the cornea of the eye. The cornea is defined by the root word "corne," which refers to this part of the eye.

- **Presbycusis.** This is a decreased hearing condition that comes on with age. It relies on the prefix "presby" and the suffix "cusis." The term "presby" means old age, and the term "cusis" refers to hearing.

- **Cycloplegic.** This is a drug, usually an eyedrop, that causes paralysis of the ciliary body of the eye. The term "cyclo" refers to the ciliary body, while "plegic" refers to the paralysis of the muscle.

- **Dacryocystitis.** This is an inflammation of the tear sac. The term "dacryocyst" means tear sac or lacrimal sac, and the suffix "itis" refers to inflammation.

- **Dacryoadenitis.** This is an inflammation of the "tear gland." The term "dacryoaden" refers to the tear gland, and "itis" refers to inflammation.

- **Fovea.** This is a pit or depression located in the retina. This is an example of something being defined by its shape as the term "fovea" means pit or depression.

- **Goniometer.** This is a device used in ophthalmology to measure the angle of head turning in the strabismus. It relies on the term "gonio," which means "angle," and "meter" means something that measures.

- **Iritis.** This is an inflammation of the colored part of the eye. It relies on the small root word "ir," which refers to iris, and "itis," which refers to an inflammation of the iris.

- **Iridectomy.** This is a surgical procedure that involves a cut in the iris. The term "irid" means iris and "ectomy" refers to the removal, excision, or resection of the iris.

- **Keratitis.** This is an inflammation of the cornea. It relies on the root word "kerat," which means cornea, and "itis," which refers to an inflammation of the cornea.

- **Lacrimal duct.** This is another word for tear duct. It makes use of the term "lacrim," which means tear duct, and the suffix "al," which means pertaining to.

- **Mydriatic.** This refers to a medication used to dilate the pupils. The root word "mydr" refers to "widening," as in widening the pupils.

- **Myringotomy tubes.** These are tubes placed in the tympanic membrane after making a cut in the membrane for the tube to fit in. The word "myring" means eardrum, or tympanic membrane, and "tomy" refers to cutting into something.

- **Oculomotor nerve.** This is one of the cranial nerves that helps run the external eye muscles. The term "oculo" refers to eye, while "motor" means movement. This is a nerve that acts in the movement of the eye.

- **Ophthalmologist.** This is a specialist in the study of the eyes. The term "ophthalmo" means eye and "ist" means specialist.

- **Hemianopsia.** This is a condition in which a person has lost vision on one side of their visual field. The prefix "hemi" means half, and the modifying root word "an" means no or not. The main root word is "opsia," which refers to vision condition.

- **Optometrist.** This is a specialist in the study of vision. The word "opto" means vision, while "metr" is a take on "meter," which means to measure. The suffix "ist" refers to specialist. This is a specialist in the measurement of vision.

- **Optical.** This refers to vision or eye. An optical illusion is something that is a "trick of the eye." The word "optico" means eye or vision.

- **Otalgia.** This is pain in the ear. The root word "ot" means ear, or pertaining to the ear, while the suffix "algia" refers to the sensation of pain.

- **Macrotia.** This basically means a large ear condition. The prefix "macr" means large, while the suffix "otia" means ear condition. It basically means to have big ears.

- **Palpebral fissure.** This is the angle of the eye opening, or the space made by opening the eyelids. It is based on the root word "palpebr," which means "eyelid," and the suffix "al," which means pertaining to.

- **Phacoemulsification.** This is a surgical procedure in which the eye's internal lens is emulsified with an ultrasonic handpiece and aspirated from the eye. The root word "phaco" means lens, identifying the place in the eye that gets emulsified.

- **Phototherapy.** This is light treatment used in the management of hyperbilirubinemia in newborns. It is based on the words for light, which is "photo," and "therapy," which means treatment.

- **Pupillary light reflex.** This is a word based on the root word "pupill," which means "pupil." The suffix "ary" means pertaining to. It is the light reflex of constriction that happens when a light is shined into the eye.

- **Retinopathy.** This is a disease of the retina. A person, for example, with diabetic retinopathy will have a diseased retina. It is based on the root word "retino," which means retina, and the suffix "pathy," which means "disease."

- **Tympanic membrane and tympanoplasty.** These are word meaning eardrum, and surgical repair of the eardrum. The root word is "tympan" or "tympano" and, in the latter case, "plasty" refers to "surgical repair."

- **Uveitis.** This is an inflammation of the uvea of the eye. The uvea is the vascular layer of the eye, and the term is based on the root word "uve" for "uvea." The suffix means inflammation.

- **Vitreous humor.** This is the aqueous humor of the eye, which is the water/liquid that gives the eye its shape. The root word "vitr" means vitreous body of the eye, and "ous" means pertaining to.

As you have seen, there are some terms that are easier to memorize than others because they are used in common English. Words related to the different parts of the eye and ear are often based on Latin and Greek terms that used the shape or appearance of the body area to define the term. Hopefully, this chapter has not been too dizzying and has given you a better understanding of the special senses of the eyes and ears.

CHAPTER 14:

THE NERVOUS SYSTEM AND PSYCHIATRY

In this chapter, the terms related to the nervous system and psychiatry are studied together. This is because there can be overlap between these two areas of medicine. Some terms will be relatively familiar, such as "anesthesia" and "coma," while others will be more difficult. This is especially true of the nervous system terms, which are less "mainstream" when compared to psychiatric terms.

Root Words in the Nervous System and Psychiatry

Here are the major root words and terms used in the study of neurology and psychiatry:

- **Alges/o.** This is the root word for sensitivity to pain.
- **Algesia.** This is the suffix term for sensitivity to pain.
- **Anxi/o.** This is the root word for anxious or uneasy.
- **Asthenia.** This is the root word for lack of strength.
- **Astro.** This is the prefix for star or star-shaped.
- **Calcul/o or Calculia.** These are root words meaning "to compute."
- **Cata.** This is the root word for down.
- **Kathisia or cathisia.** These are suffix terms meaning "sitting."
- **Caus/o.** This is the root word meaning burning or to burn.
- **Cerebell/o.** This is the root word for cerebellum (the back part of the brain).
- **Cerebr/o.** This is the root word for cerebrum (the largest portion of the brain).
- **Comat/o.** This is the root word that means "deep sleep."

- **Coma.** This is the suffix meaning "deep sleep."
- **Dur/o.** This is the root word for dura mater.
- **Dynia.** This is a suffix word that means "pain."
- **Encephal/o.** This is the root word that means "brain."
- **Equin/o.** This is the root word that means "horse."
- **Erg/o.** This is the root word that means work.
- **Esthes/o.** This is a root word meaning nervous sensation.
- **Enthesi/o.** This is another root word meaning nervous sensation.
- **Esthesia.** This is a suffix term meaning nervous sensation.
- **Ganglion/o.** This is the root word that means ganglion, or a collection of nerve cell bodies.
- **Gli/o.** This is the root word that means neuroglial cells or glial cells.
- **Gnos/o.** This is the root word for knowledge.
- **Hallucin/o.** This is the root word for hallucination.
- **Hypn/o.** This is the root word for sleep.
- **Hypophys/o.** This is the root word for pituitary gland.
- **Hypothalm/o.** This is the root word for hypothalamus.
- **Ideo.** This is the root word meaning idea or mental images.
- **Idi/o.** This is the root word for unknown, individual, or distinct.
- **Lal/o or lalia.** This is the root word for babble or speech.
- **Lemma.** This is a suffix word meaning covering or sheath.
- **Lepsy.** This is a suffix term meaning seizure.
- **Leptic.** This is a suffix word meaning to seize or take hold of.
- **Lex/o.** This is a root word that means word or phrase.
- **Lexia.** This is a suffix word that means word or phrase.
- **Lob/o.** This is a root word meaning lobe, as in the lobe of the brain.
- **Mania.** This is a suffix the means obsessive preoccupation.
- **Medull/o.** This is a root word that means medulla (inner section), middle, or soft

marrow.

- **Mening/o.** This is a root word for meninges (the covering of the brain and spinal cord).

- **Meningi/o.** This is a root word for meninges as well.

- **Mnesia.** This is a suffix that means memory.

- **Narc/o.** This is a root word meaning sleep or stupor.

- **Neur/o.** This is a root word for nerve.

- **Noc/i.** This is a root word meaning to cause harm, pain, or injury.

- **Noia.** This is a suffix word for will or mind.

- **Paresis.** This is a suffix word meaning weakness.

- **Phob/o.** This is a root word that means fear.

- **Phobia.** This is a suffix term meaning fear.

- **Phori/a.** This is a root word that means to bear, carry, or have a feeling/mental state.

- **Plegia.** This is a suffix term meaning palsy or paralysis.

- **Plegia.** This is a suffix term meaning paralysis or palsy.

- **Plex/o.** This is a root word meaning plexus, or a network of nerves.

- **Praxia.** This is a suffix term that means "action."

- **Psych/o.** This is a major root word meaning "mind."

- **Receptor or ceptor.** These are suffix words that mean receiver.

- **Schiz/o.** This is a root word meaning "split."

- **Somn/o.** This is a root word meaning sleep.

- **Somnia.** This is a root word meaning sleep and is often used as a suffix.

- **Thalam/o.** This is the root word for "thalamus."

- **Thymia.** This is a suffix meaning condition of the mind.

- **Thymic.** This is a suffix meaning pertaining to the mind.

- **Trem/o or tremul/o.** This is a root word that means tremor or shaking.

- **Vag/o.** This is the root word for the vagus nerve.

Putting it All Together

These are the terms used in real-life settings; we have included them in order to help you see what words are used in medicine that make use of root words and suffixes. Here are some added prefixes and suffixes to further help define such terms:

- **Analgesia.** This means something that decreases the sensitivity to pain. For example, the word "an" means no, not, or without, and "algesia" is the suffix term for sensitivity to pain. An analgesic also decreases pain and makes use of the root word "alges."

- **Anxiolytic.** This is a word that usually refers to a medication that reduces anxiety. The root word is "anxio," which means anxious or uneasy, while "lytic" means to reduce, destroy, separate, or breakdown.

- **Neurasthenia.** This is a medical term used for people who have nervous exhaustion or nervous weakness. It uses the root word "neur" for "nerve," and the suffix "asthenia" for weakness or lack of strength.

- **Astrocytoma.** This is a brain cancer that is star-shaped. It is named for "astro," which means star-shaped, and "cyt," which means cell. The suffix "oma" refers to a tumor.

- **Acalculia.** This is a psychiatric and neurologic term referring to someone who has lost the ability to do math problems or to compute things. It is based on the prefix "a" for no and the suffix "calculia" for "to compute."

- **Cataplexy.** This is a condition where a patient suddenly loses muscle tone and falls down. It is based on the root word "cata," which means "down," and the ending "plexy," which means "nerves" or a network of nerves.

- **Akathisia.** This is a neuropsychiatric term referring to someone who has a condition where they can't sit still. The term "a" is combined with the suffix "kathisia," which means sitting, implying that the person cannot sit still.

- **Causalgia.** This is a condition in which the person has burning pain in their extremities. The root word is "caus," which means burning, and the suffix "algia," refers to "pain."

- **Cerebellopontine angle.** This is a brain structure related to the cerebellum and the pons. The term "cerebello" is in there because of the relationship to the cerebellum.

- **Cerebrum.** This is the largest part of the brain and is the structure that is named for the root word "cerebro," which refers to it.

- **Comatose.** This refers to "one who is in a deep sleep." The phrase "comato" refers to deep sleep.

- **Coma.** This is simple as the root word for this is the same as the term. Basically, it refers to being in a deep sleep.

- **Subdural hematoma.** This is a collection of blood beneath the dura mater. The term "sub" means beneath, while the root word "dur" means dura mater, and the suffix "al" means pertaining to. The word "hematoma" basically means "blood tumor" — even though this is not technically a tumor in the true sense of the word.

- **Encephalopathy.** This means a disease of the brain. The root word "encephalo" means brain, while the word "pathy" means "disease of."

- **Cauda equina.** This refers to a tuft of the spinal cord that is shaped like the tail of the horse. The word uses the term for horse, which is "equin."

- **Ergonomic.** This refers to something that is easier to work with because of its structure. The term "ergo" is used to describe work, while the term "nom" means custom.

- **Anesthesia.** This is a practice of relieving a person of their nervous sensation. The prefix "an" means no or not, while the suffix "esthesia" refers to nervous sensation. Other related root words are "esthesia" and "enthesio" — both of which refer to nervous sensation.

- **Neuroglial cells.** These are supporting cells in the brain. They use the root word "gli," which means "glial cell."

- **Agnosia.** This literally means "no knowledge." It involves an inability to interpret sensations and hence to recognize things, typically as a result of brain damage. The root word is "gnos" and the prefix is "a" for "no or not."

- **Hallucination.** This is seeing or hearing something that isn't there. The obvious root word for this is "hallucin." There is also the term "hallucinogenic," which is a drug that causes a person to hallucinate.

- **Hypnosis.** This involves causing a person to go into a state that mimics sleep. A hypnagogic hallucination happens when a person is sleeping. Both use the root word "hypn," which means "sleep."

- **Hypophyseal fossa**. This is a depression on the upper surface of the sphenoid bone, lodging in the pituitary gland. The root word is "hypophys/o," which means pituitary gland, and is what the fossa is named after.

- **Hypothalamic**. This refers to the hypothalamus and is based on the root word "hypothalam," which means "hypothalamus."

- **Idiopathic**. This is a disease that has no obvious origin. The root word is "idio," which means unknown, individual, or distinct. The suffix "pathic" means referring to a disease state.

- **Echolalia**. This means the meaningless repetition of another person's spoken words as a symptom of a psychiatric disorder. The root words are "echo," which means reflected sound and "lalia," which means babble or speech.

- **Neurilemma**. This is a sheath surrounding a nerve. It is based on the root word "neuro" for nerve and "lemma," which means sheath. The definition is the thin sheath around a nerve axon (including myelin where this is present).

- **Narcolepsy**. This is a sudden attack or "seizure" in which the patient suddenly drops and falls asleep without warning. It is based on the root word "narco," which means sleep or stupor, and the suffix "lepsy," which means seizure.

- **Neuroleptic**. This is a drug used in medicine to manage psychiatric problems. It relates to the root words "neuro" for "nerve" and "leptic" for "seize or take hold of."

- **Alexia**. This is a neurological problem in which the patient can't recognize words or phrases (the written word). It is based on the prefix "a," which means "no or not," and "lexia," which means "word or phrase." These combine to mean "no word or phrase."

- **Frontal lobe**. This is one of the lobes of the brain, of which there are several different ones. It is based on the root word "lob," which simply means "lobe."

- **Pyromania**. This is a word meaning to have an obsessive preoccupation with setting fires. The term "pyro" refers to fires, while "mania" refers to an obsessive preoccupation with something.

- **Medulla oblongata**. This is a brain structure in the middle of the brain stem. It is based on the root word "medull," which means medulla or inner section (middle).

- **Meningomyelocele.** This is a birth defect in which the spinal canal and the backbone don't close before the baby is born. It is a type of spina bifida. The root word "meningo" means "meninges," while the root word "myelo" means "spinal cord."

- **Meningeal.** This means pertaining to the meninges and comes from the root word for meninges, which is "meningi."

- **Amnesia.** This basically means "no memory." It is based on the prefix "a," which means "no or not," and "mnesia," which means memory. Patients with amnesia have no memory.

- **Nociceptor.** This is a sensory receptor that senses pain. It is based on the root word for pain, which is "noci," and the root word for receiver, which is "ceptor."

- **Paranoia.** This is a state of mind in which the patient believes people are about to harm them or mean them harm. It is based on the root word "para," which means near, beside, abnormal, apart from, or along the side of, and the root word "noia," which means mind. In this case, it means "abnormal mind."

- **Hemiparesis.** This basically means "half weakness" and refers to a state in which half of the body has, because of an injury or stroke, developed paralysis or weakness. The prefix "hemi" means "half," while the term "paresis" means "weakness."

- **Homophobia.** This is a person who is fearful of homosexuality. Literally, the term means "same fear" or the fear of someone interested in the same sex or gender.

- **Euphoria.** This literally means "good mental state." The prefix "eu" means good or normal, while "phoria" means feeling or mental state.

- **Hemiplegia.** This is a term that means "half paralysis." It is a neurological condition in which half of the body is paralyzed. It usually comes from having a stroke on one side of the brain.

- **Neuropraxia.** This basically means a transient conduction block of motor or sensory function without nerve degeneration, although loss of motor function is the most common finding. It is based on the root word "neuro" for "nerve" and "praxia" for "action," as mostly the motor nerve action is affected.

- **Psychotherapy**. This basically means "mind treatment"; the two root words are "psycho" for "mind" and "therapy" for treatment. It is talk therapy done for many types of mental conditions.

- **Schizophrenia**. This is a psychotic disorder that makes use of the root word "schizo," which means "split." "Phren" means "mind and "ia" means condition of. Literally, this means a "condition of the split mind."

- **Polysomnography**. This is a type of testing that records the patient's brain waves, the oxygen level in their blood, heart rate, and breathing, as well as eye and leg movements during a sleep study. It is based on "poly" for "many," as many things are assessed, and the root word "somno," which means "sleep." The term "graphy" refers to the "process of recording."

- **Insomnia**. This is a condition that involves not being able to get restful sleep. Basically, it means "not sleep," since "in" can mean "not." The suffix "somnia" refers to sleep.

- **Dysthymia**. This is a mildly depressed state. The term "dys" means bad, painful, difficult, or abnormal, while "thymia" refers to a condition of the mind. A related word is "thymic," which also means a condition of the mind.

- **Tremulous**. This is a word that means tremors or shaking. It is based on the root word "tremulo," which means shaking and "ous," which means pertaining to.

- **Vagus nerve.** This is a main parasympathetic nerve in the chest and abdomen. It is based on the root word "vag," which means the vagus nerve.

CHAPTER 15:

THE INTEGUMENTARY SYSTEM

The integumentary system involves the study of the skin. There are just a few root words to memorize so, compared to other chapters, this should be simpler to study. The terms also represent medical root words that apply to the fatty tissue and nails in order to round out your knowledge of skin and soft tissues.

Terms to Remember

These are the root words related to the skin that you have to memorize. Some will be very familiar, such as the root word for "cutaneous," which means pertaining to the skin, and "dermatology," which is the study of skin. Let's take a look:

- **Adip or Adipo.** These are the root words for fat or fatty tissue.
- **Cutane or Cutaneo.** These are both root words for skin.
- **Derm or Dermo.** These are root words for skin.
- **Dermat or Dermato.** These are root words for skin.
- **Hidr or Hidro.** These are both root words for sweat gland. They are both similar to "hydro," which means water.
- **Kerat/o.** This means hard and is used in words relating to the skin, hair, and nails.
- **Lip or Lipo.** These are root words for fat or fatty tissue.
- **Onych or Onycho.** These refer to the nails of the fingers or toes.
- **Plasia.** This is a suffix and refers to the formation or "growth of."
- **Prurio or Pruritis.** This is a term meaning "to itch."

- **Purpura.** This is a medical term meaning purple.

- **Seb/o or Seb/i.** This relates to sebum or "skin oil."

- **Steat/o.** This is a root word meaning fat.

- **Stear/o.** This is another root word meaning fat.

- **Trich/o or Trich/i.** This is a root word meaning hair.

- **Xanth/o.** This is a root word meaning yellow.

- **Xero.** This is a root word or prefix meaning "dry."

Putting it All Together

Despite the fewness of terms that have to be memorized in this chapter, there are many different words that can be made from them. Let's look at a few of them so you can see how to combine these root words with the prefixes and suffixes you have come to know well:

- **Xerosis.** This is a term that means an abnormal amount of dryness. In the skin, it means "to have very dry skin."

- **Xanthoma.** This is a small skin lump (remember that "oma" means tumor) that is yellow and made from cholesterol. It is not actually a tumor, but is instead a collection of cholesterol.

- **Hypertrichosis.** This can be divided into "hyper/trich/osis" and means a condition of excessive amounts of hair. People with this condition have hair all over their body.

- **Stearic acid.** This is a fatty acid using the term based on "stear," which means fatty, plus the ending "ic," which means "pertaining to."

- **Steatorrhea.** This is actually a GI term, which means to have fat in the stool. It is based on the root word "steat/o," which means fat, and the suffix "rrhea," which means "to flow."

- **Purpura.** This is a root word meaning "purple" and refers to purplish bruised areas of the skin, or a "purplish rash."

- **Dysplasia.** This means the abnormal growth of something. It makes use of the prefix "dys," which means bad, and "plasia," which means "the growth of." This is used throughout medical terminology to represent many precancerous conditions.

- **Onychomycosis.** This is divided into "onycho/myc/osis" and means the condition, or disease of, a fungal infection of the nail. There are two root words in this term: "onycho" or "nail" and "myc" or "fungus."

- **Lipodystrophy.** This term breaks down into "lipo/dys/trophy," which is an abnormal distribution of fat in the body. It is based on the root word for "fat" and the terms "dys" (or bad/abnormal) and "trophy," which refers to "a condition of nutrition or growth."

- **Hyperhidrosis.** This word breaks down into "hyper/hidr/osis" and is an abnormal condition of excessive sweating. It is based on the common prefix "hyper," which means too much, the root word "hidr," which means "sweat," and "osis," or the abnormal condition of or "excessive amount of" something.

- **Cutaneous.** This means "related to skin" and is based on the root word for skin, "cutane." Interestingly, the drug Accutane is a skin drug for acne that also uses this root word.

- **Dermatosis.** This is an abnormal condition of the skin and is based on the root word for skin, "dermato."

As promised, this chapter wasn't too hard. Many terms were easily recognizable and, because your memory for common prefixes and suffixes is probably getting better, you likely have a good idea of the meaning of the word (the category of word you are looking at) before you actually get to the meaning of the root word.

CHAPTER 16:

TERMS RELATED TO BODY STRUCTURES AND ORGANIZATION

No study of anatomy would be complete without understanding the positional terms that describe where things are located. When naming two different structures, anatomists centuries ago used specific terminology to identify the "superior" structure and the "inferior" structure or the "proximal" versus the "distal" structure. Knowing these terms helps the student recognize the position of two structures as they exist in relationship to one another.

The key directional terms are these:

- **Superior.** This refers to anything closer to the head. There is, for example, the superior mesenteric artery, which refers to the artery in the abdomen that is closer to the head than the "inferior" mesenteric artery.

- **Inferior.** This refers to anything closer to the caudal end of the body. When talking about caudal, it is not the same thing as being closer to the feet; instead this means closer to the buttocks or the bottom of the torso. The inferior vena cava is a major vein below the level of the heart that is closer to the bottom of the torso than the superior vena cava, which is closer to the head.

- **Posterior.** This describes something that is closer to the back of something. In humans, it refers to the back of the body, whether it be the torso, arms, legs, or head. For example, the posterior pituitary gland is located closer to the back of the head than the anterior pituitary gland.

- **Anterior.** This describes something closer to the front of something. In the human body, it refers to something located nearer to the front of the body, whether it be the torso, arms, legs, or head. For example, the anterior superior iliac crest defines a part of the pelvic bone structure that is both anterior and superior when compared to the rest of the pelvic bone.

- **Lateral.** This refers to something that is closer to the side of the body and is in direct opposition to the term "medial." The lateral malleolus is the bony prominence on the outside of the ankle and is differentiated from the medial malleolus, which is located on the inside of the ankle.

- **Medial.** This is the term used to describe something located more to the middle or midline of the body. It can be in the torso, arms, legs, or head. The medial meniscus is the portion of the cartilage in the knee that is located on the inside portion of the knee. The designation "medial" is used to distinguish it from the lateral meniscus on the outside of the knee.

- **Deep.** This refers to something located further away from the skin when compared to something that is superficial (or close to the skin surface). The deep circumflex iliac artery and vein are located deeper to the skin than other arteries and veins in the iliac artery. It can be expected to be located relatively further away than more superficial structures.

- **Superficial.** This refers to something close to the surface of the body or the skin of the body. For example, the condition of "superficial thrombophlebitis" refers to an inflammation of the superficial veins of the body (close to the skin). These can be differentiated from "deep vein thrombosis," which represents deeper vein blood clots, usually in the leg.

- **Proximal.** This is a relational term that defines something closer to a particular reference point, usually the center of the body. For example, the proximal tibia is the part of the tibia bone that is closer to the center of the body than any portion of the tibia further away from the center of the body.

- **Distal.** This refers to something further away from the center of the body when compared to some other reference point. It is essentially the opposite of the term "proximal." The distal tibia is further away from the center of the body than the proximal tibia.

- **Dorsal.** This term can be used instead of posterior and means the back side of something or the upper side. The dorsal fin of a fish is located on the upper/back part of its body (as opposed to a ventral fin).

- **Ventral.** This refers to something anterior in the body. It can also mean the lower aspect of the body (especially when referring to a four-legged animal). In humans, a ventral hernia is, by definition, located on the abdomen, in the front part of the body.

- **Cranial.** This can also mean something superior and basically refers to something close to the head. There are numerous cranial nerves, which are labeled as such because they originate from the head and travel to the face and neck without having to travel down the spinal cord. The "cranium" is another term for the skull that encloses the brain.

- **Caudal.** This term is the opposite of cranial and refers to something close to the bottom of the torso. The medical diagnosis of "cauda equina syndrome" refers to a lesion affecting the cauda equina, which is the most inferior/distal part of the spinal column. Caudal, in humans, refers to being close to the feet. The term, "caudad," refers to something close to the feet. In embryology, it refers to something close to the tail and, in animals, it refers to something close to the tail or hind part of the body.

- **Horizontal.** There really aren't any anatomic terms linked to the term "horizontal," but it can be used to describe any plane that passes through the standing body that is parallel to the floor.

- **Anteroposterior or Posteroanterior.** This refers to directionality. An AP anteroposterior X-ray is one that sends X-rays from the front to the back of the body. A PA chest X-ray is the opposite to this as it involves X-rays that travel from the back to the front of the chest.

- **Inferolateral and inferomedial.** This refers to something that is both inferior in the body and either lateral (to the side) or medial (to the center) of the body. It is used to describe something in reference to another point on the body.

- **Pronation.** This is a movement term and refers to a rotation of the forearm and hand so that the palm of the hand is down or posterior. It also refers to the movement of the ankle and foot so that the bottom of the foot is rotated inward. Rather than an anatomical term, it refers mostly to the physiological movement of the extremity. The term "pronate" is the actual action taking place.

- **Supination.** This is a movement term as well and refers to a rotation of the forearm and hand so that the palm of the hand is up or anterior. It can also refer to the movement of the foot and ankle so that the bottom of the foot is rotated outward.

- **Adduction.** This is a movement term that refers to any motion of an extremity that is traveling toward the body. It can be an arm or a leg in humans.

- **Abduction.** This is a movement term that refers to any motion of an extremity that is traveling away from the body. It can be an arm or a leg in humans.

- **Prone and Supine.** These are static terms that refer to the position of the body. Prone is lying face down (in a human), while supine is lying face up (in humans).

- **Vertical.** This refers to any line in the body that is perpendicular to the floor in an upright person. It is the opposite of a horizontal line.

Body Planes

In defining the anatomical position of things, there are a few body planes that are defined and made use of. These planes are used in medical imaging, in the study of embryology, and in describing certain body movements. These include the following:

- **Transverse Plane.** This can mean any plane that divides the human body into inferior and superior parts. It is a line that is both parallel to the floor and perpendicular to the upright human spine. This is also referred to as the XZ plane.

- **Sagittal Plane.** This is any imaginary line that is parallel to the median plane. The median plane is the line that divides the body into the right (dexter) and left (sinister) sides. The sagittal plane does not have to be directly dividing the body into a left and right half, but it is always parallel to the median plane. The sagittal plane is also called the YZ plane or the lateral plane.

- **Coronal Plane.** This is a vertical line in the human body that is perpendicular to the floor and divides the body into anterior/ventral (abdominal) and posterior (dorsum, or back of the body) sections. The coronal plane is also called the frontal plane or the XY plane in the body.

Any plane perpendicular to the transverse plane is considered a longitudinal plane. The sagittal plane, any parasagittal plane (a line parallel to the sagittal plane), and the coronal plane are all considered longitudinal planes because they are all perpendicular to the transverse line/plane.

The body planes are particularly important in medical imaging, such as PET scanning, MRI scanning, CT scanning, and ultrasonography. The radiologist places the body in an XYZ axis in order to identify/locate the position of bodily organs. It is used for therapeutic radiology, in which the X-rays are used to target a tumor in a specific part of the body.

Body Cavities

All vertebrates have fluid-filled spaces that are referred to as the body cavities. The different body cavities contain all of the organs in the body. There are body cavities for all the major organ systems of the body. Some body cavities have membranes that divide them and separate them from other body cavities. For example, the meninges are the tissues that separate the dorsal cavity organs (the nervous system) from the rest of the body.

The mesothelium is a tissue type that holds the ventral cavity. Sub-tissue types that make up the mesothelium are the pleural lining (pleura) of the lungs, the peritoneum of the abdominopelvic cavity, and the pericardium, which holds the heart.

A body cavity is any fluid-filled space in a vertebrate or any multicellular organism. It refers specifically to the space where the internal organs are kept. When referencing the human body cavity, the ventral cavity is what people are referring to, as it is the biggest body cavity (although there are several others). The blood and its vessels are not located in one specific cavity, but travel through all the cavities.

The different body cavities are these:

- **Dorsal cavity.** The dorsal cavity is located on the dorsal aspect of the body and houses the organs of the central nervous system, including the spinal cord and brain. It is covered by the meninges, which is a many-layered membrane.

- **Cranial cavity.** This is the entirety of the space inside the skull and is the uppermost part of the dorsal cavity. It contains the cerebrospinal fluid, the brain, and the meninges (meningeal lining).

- **Vertebral cavity.** This is the lowermost aspect of the dorsal cavity and contains the structures inside the vertebral column. It includes the meningeal tissues around the spinal cord, the spinal cord itself, and the fluid around the spinal cord. It is the narrowest body cavity and it runs up and down.

- **Ventral cavity.** This is the largest of all the body cavities and contains a variety of organ systems, known as the viscera of the body. The ventral cavity has anterior (upper) and posterior (lower) parts that are divided by the diaphragm, a large muscular structure beneath the lungs.

- **Thoracic cavity.** This is the anterior or upper part of the ventral cavity that is contained nearly entirely by the rib cage. It contains most of the organs of the respiratory system and the organs of the cardiovascular system, as well as a few other organs, such as the thymus gland and the esophagus. It is lined by two different kinds of mesothelium: the pleural lining (pleura) of the lungs, and the pericardium (which contains the heart and part of the major vessels).

- **Abdominopelvic.** This is the posterior, or lower part, of the ventral cavity located beneath the diaphragm. It contains the abdominal and pelvic organs. It is subdivided into the pelvic cavity and the abdominal cavity. The abdominal cavity is not covered by bone and contains the digestive organs, renal organs, and a few other organs, such as the adrenal glands (part of the endocrine system). The pelvic cavity is beneath the abdominal cavity and is housed within the pelvic bone structures. It contains part of the genitourinary system (the bladder, mainly) and the entirety of the reproductive system. The lining of the abdominopelvic cavity is the peritoneum, a type of mesothelium.

Abdominal Quadrants and Areas

The abdomen is a large cavity with organs from several different physiological body areas. There are four quadrants to the abdomen and nine different regions or areas. The regions are smaller than the quadrants. The perineum (or area of the body containing the genitals) is sometimes considered to be the tenth abdominal region.

The main purpose of the different abdominal regions and quadrants is to have some method of describing the regional abdominal anatomy and to distinguish (based on the patient's pain) the diseased organs which may be causing the patient to feel a certain pain.

The other purpose of having regions and quadrants in the abdomen is so that anatomists have a method of discussing the various anatomical structures in the study of anatomy. Anatomists can describe in detail which organs are in which regions of the abdomen, and they can expect certain organs to remain relatively fixed in a specific region.

The Quadrants of the Abdomen

As mentioned, there are four different quadrants in the abdomen, which are defined according to an intersection between the median/sagittal plane and one of the transverse planes. These include the following:

- **Left Lower Quadrant**. This is, of course, in the left lower region of the abdomen. It contains the vast majority of the small intestines, some of the large intestine (mainly the descending colon), the left-sided female reproductive organs, and the left-sided ureter. This means that it is part of the GI tract, genitourinary tract, and reproductive tract. If a patient has pain in this area, colitis or diverticulitis are typical causes. In females, possible causes for pain in this area also include pelvic inflammatory disease, endometriosis, or a ruptured left ovarian cyst.

- **Right lower Quadrant.** This is the abdominal quadrant that contains the cecum, appendix, part of the small intestines, part of the ascending colon, the right-sided female organs (such as the right ovary), and the right ureter. Common underlying problems with right lower quadrant abdominal pain include appendicitis and, in females, right ovarian cyst rupture or endometriosis of the right side of the pelvis.

- **Right upper quadrant.** This part of the abdomen contains most of the liver, the gallbladder, a small part of the stomach, the right kidney, the ascending and part of the transverse colon, and a portion of the small intestines. Pain in the right upper quadrant is most related to the liver and gallbladder, although (in rare cases) the stomach can also have pain here.

- **Left upper quadrant.** The left upper quadrant houses a small portion of the liver, the stomach (most of it), the spleen, the pancreas, the left kidney, and parts of the small intestine, transverse colon, and descending colon. Pain in this area of the abdomen would most likely be secondary to stomach ulcers, or malrotation of the

139

small intestine or colon.

Nine Abdominal Divisions

There are nine regions to the abdominopelvic region that can be used to identify places for things inside the abdomen or pelvis. They are marked by two parasagittal planes and two transverse planes that are on either side, and above and below the navel. Most organs can be found in more than one region, but the regions are still helpful for anatomists to define the various areas of this large cavity. There is no coronal variation in this region, only parasagittal and transverse planes.

The nine regions of the abdominopelvic cavity include the following:

- **Right hypochondriac.** This is the upper right section of the abdomen and contains the gallbladder, the right side of the liver, the right kidney, and some of the small intestine.

- **Left hypochondriac.** This region contains most of the spleen, the left kidney, the pancreas, part of the colon, and part of the stomach.

- **Epigastric.** This is the main region for the stomach, but it also contains part of the liver, duodenum, part of the pancreas, part of the spleen, and the left adrenal gland.

- **Right lumbar.** This is where the gallbladder, the left kidney, the ascending colon, and part of the liver are located.

- **Left lumbar.** This is where the descending colon, part of the spleen, and the left kidney are located. Pyelonephritis of the left kidney would give pain in this area of the abdomen.

- **Umbilical.** This is the centermost aspect of the abdomen and is located around the navel. It contains much of the duodenum, ileum, and jejunum. It also contains the transverse colon (which connects the ascending and descending colon) and the bottom portions of both kidneys.

- **Right iliac.** This is the region where the appendix, right iliac fossa, and the cecum would be located, and would also be where pain that is secondary to a ruptured appendix would be located.

- **Left iliac.** This contains a portion of the descending colon, the left iliac fossa, and the sigmoid colon. It is also referred to as the left inguinal region.

- **Hypogastric.** The term "hypogastric" means below the stomach, and it contains those organs just above the pubic symphysis. It includes the bladder, part of the sigmoid colon, the anus, and the reproductive organs.

CHAPTER 17:

CONCLUSION

Let's take a moment to take in the enormity of the language you've just learned. In truth, the study of medical terminology is like learning a new language; there are innumerable terms that everyone in healthcare should know—or at least have a good idea of what they mean. Most represent medical terms that were first created in the Greek and Roman times, when the Greek and Latin languages were used to create them. Even terms that have recently been defined in medicine have stayed true to these ancient words that first defined medicine as we know it today.

Over time, you have probably noticed that, while there are many prefixes and suffixes, they are repeated over and over again—so they will easily become ingrained in your memory. This is a good thing because you refer to them first when defining and creating medical terms. It's only last that you look at the root word (or root words) in order to glean the area of the body being discussed.

The latter chapters of the book are challenging because each one defines a whole new set of terms that pertain exclusively to the area of the body being covered. Unfortunately, the root words are, for the most part, unique, so they have to be memorized. The good news is that they reinforce the prefixes and suffixes over and over again so you can better commit them to memory.

This brings us back to the introduction and to the advice we've already talked about. If you have time to make flashcards out of index cards (cut in half if possible), you can play the "medical terminology game" by yourself. This is a type of solitaire that gets easier over time because, after you've truly memorized a term and have proven that to yourself, you can take the card out of the pile. What's left over will gradually shrink until you have memorized everything.

But can you actually memorize everything? With the information in this book and a set of flashcards, it is definitely possible. Having knowledge of the prefixes, suffixes, and root words will serve you well in your medical endeavors and will make you a more valuable member of your medical team. Nothing will stand in your way of knowing what a medical specialist is trying to convey to you or what you're reading in a medical journal. Your newfound knowledge will open up a new world for you as you continue on your never-ending quest for the latest in medical information. The best of luck to you!!

Made in the USA
Middletown, DE
19 March 2021